28-Day Body Shapeover

Brad Schoenfeld

HUMAN KINETICS

Library of Congress Cataloging-in-Publication Data

Schoenfeld, Brad, 1962-
  28-day body shapeover / Brad Schoenfeld.
    p. cm.
  Includes index.
  ISBN 0-7360-6045-6 (soft cover)
  1. Physical fitness--Handbooks, manuals, etc. 2. Exercise--Handbooks, manuals, etc. I. Title:
Twenty-eight day body shapeover. II. Title.
  GV481.S275 2006
  613.7'1--dc22
                                    2005025188

ISBN: 0-7360-6045-6

The Web addresses cited in this text were current as of October 2005, unless otherwise noted.

Acquisitions Editor: Martin Barnard; **Developmental Editor:** Kase Johnstun; **Assistant Editor:**
Cory Weber; **Copyeditor:** PagePerfect Editorial Services; **Proofreader:** Bethany J. Bentley; **Indexer:**
Marie Rizzo; **Graphic Designer:** Nancy Rasmus; **Graphic Artist:** Tara Welsch; **Photo Manager:**
Dan Wendt; **Cover Designer:** Keith Blomberg; **Photographer (cover):** Terry Wild; **Photographer
(interior):** Photos on pages 58 and 121 of Machine Rear Lateral and on pages 66 and 193 of Cable
High Pulley Crossover by Terry Wild; all other photos by Dan Wendt; **Printer:** United Graphics

We thank New York Sports Club in Croton-on-Hudson, New York, for assistance in providing the
location for the photo shoot for this book.

Human Kinetics books are available at special discounts for bulk purchase. Special editions or book
excerpts can also be created to specification. For details, contact the Special Sales Manager at Human
Kinetics.

Printed in the United States of America   10   9   8   7   6   5   4   3   2   1

Human Kinetics
Web site: www.HumanKinetics.com

United States: Human Kinetics
P.O. Box 5076
Champaign, IL 61825-5076
800-747-4457
e-mail: humank@hkusa.com

Canada: Human Kinetics
475 Devonshire Road Unit 100
Windsor, ON N8Y 2L5
800-465-7301 (in Canada only)
e-mail: orders@hkcanada.com

Europe: Human Kinetics
107 Bradford Road
Stanningley
Leeds LS28 6AT, United Kingdom
+44 (0) 113 255 5665
e-mail: hk@hkeurope.com

Australia: Human Kinetics
57A Price Avenue
Lower Mitcham, South Australia 5062
08 8277 1555
e-mail: liaw@hkaustralia.com

New Zealand: Human Kinetics
Division of Sports Distributors NZ Ltd.
P.O. Box 300 226 Albany
North Shore City
Auckland
0064 9 448 1207
e-mail: info@humankinetics.co.nz

28-Day Body Shapeover

Contents

Preface

Here in the United States, the quest to be lean and fit has become a national obsession. In our pursuit to achieve the ultimate body, we seem willing to try almost anything to see results. Moreover, impatience is the norm rather than the exception; we don't just want a better body—we want it *now!*

Not surprisingly, scores of hucksters have attempted to capitalize on the "get buff quick" craze. From fancy exercise gizmos to magic pills, creams, and potions, people spend billions each year on products claiming to zap the fat and pack on the muscle quickly and easily. Sadly, these products never work as advertised, leaving those who fall prey to their clever marketing tactics hopelessly frustrated (as well as lighter in the wallet).

With all the bogus cure-alls out there, many women are turning to surgery to solve their body image woes. According to a recent study by the American Society of Plastic Surgeons, one-third of the population is currently contemplating some sort of cosmetic procedure and more than a million Americans will actually take the plunge and undergo the knife in 2005 alone. Upper arm lifts, breast lifts, tummy tucks, liposuction—the list of options reads like a high-tech cosmetic menu. But surgery has numerous drawbacks. It is costly and painful, there is often unsightly scarring, and the results are temporary unless accompanied by lifestyle changes. In some cases, botched surgical procedures have even resulted in death!

Fortunately, you don't have to resort to worthless fitness-in-a-bottle potions or expensive, risky surgical procedures to achieve a great body in a relatively short period of time. If you have the will, this book will show you the way.

In the pages within, I have detailed my time-tested program designed to noticeably improve your appearance in just one month's time. This is not a gimmick-based, quick-fix scheme but rather a tried and true formula for success based on my extensive scientific research and more than fifteen years of experience as a nationally recognized fitness and nutritional expert.

The exercise program is a modified version of my acclaimed High-Energy Fitness system of training, designed to simultaneously increase muscle while shedding body fat. Focusing on the concept of quality over quantity, it is extremely time efficient, requiring only 30 minutes of exercise per session. The intensive nature of the program will maximize a phenomenon called *excess postexercise oxygen consumption*—the amount of calories burned after the completion of a workout—heightening fat burning for almost two full days following a training session! And for those who can't get to a gym, I've included a full complement of home-based alternatives that require minimal equipment.

The nutritional regimen is based on the concept of *set point* (the predetermined amount of fat that the body strives to maintain), which employs a strategy that fools the body into believing it needs to maintain less fat than it is genetically programmed to store. Not only does it help to reduce body fat as low as possible, but, more importantly, it allows you to keep it off over the long term. And unlike many other diets, it is not restrictive, allowing consumption of all the major food groups, which in turn improves adherence to the program. There is even a regimented *refeed day*, where you'll get to indulge in all of your favorite sin foods, helping to satisfy cravings and prevent bingeing.

The heart of the book is a four-week, calendar-style routine that is laid out in chronological order for ease of use. Starting with Day 1 and ending with Day 28, it takes all the guesswork out of developing a fitness regimen. Every exercise, every set, every rep, every morsel of food is spelled out in detail. All you have to do is turn to the page for that particular day, and you'll know exactly what to do!

Here's what you can expect to achieve by following the program as outlined over the four-week period:

- A safe and healthy loss of 6 to 8 pounds of body fat
- A 2- to 4-pound increase in lean muscle tissue
- A 50 percent increase in absolute strength
- A noticeable improvement in energy levels, endurance, and posture
- *And more . . .*

All this in just one month's time! And better yet, results can be enhanced by following the program over a longer time frame. In fact, in just three short months you can completely transform your appearance, achieving results that are sure to turn heads.

Ideally, it will help if you've had some previous training experience. Those who are intermediate to advanced exercisers will be able to go full force from the onset, taking maximal advantage of the metabolic boost that high-energy training provides. Beginners will need to tone down the intensity a bit in order to acclimate the body to the intense demands of the program, but a beginner will still reap superior rewards over time. Either way, you should be ecstatic with the change in mind, body, and spirit.

In sum, the revolutionary program I've used on thousands of women in my private training facility can now be yours simply by reading this book and heeding its advice. If you put in the effort, success is all but guaranteed!

Acknowledgments

To my agent, Bob Silverstein, for making sure that this project found the proper home. Your guidance is always appreciated.

To Martin Barnard for seeing the potential in this project. Your expert editorial suggestions were right on the money.

To Kase Johnstun for helping to develop this project to its fullest potential despite some bumps in the road.

To Gina Giuliano, Clarissa Chueire, and Lisa Vacarelli for demonstrating exercise form to perfection. You are true fitness models.

To all my clients, past and present, at the Personal Training Center for Women for being an inspiration for this program.

To Terry Kowalski for use of the terrific facilities at the New York Sports Club.

28-Day Body Shapeover

Before beginning my 28-Day Shapeover plan, it is essential to understand the protocols that make up its foundation. In this chapter, you'll learn the science behind my fitness philosophy, providing all the ammunition necessary to achieve your physique goals. Once you get familiar with the concepts presented herein, you'll be able to dive headfirst into the program; a better body is only four weeks away!

Shapeover Exercise

It never ceases to amaze me how many women ignore exercise when they are trying to lose weight. They'll go on some ultra-low-calorie diet and literally starve themselves to thinness; their main form of activity consists of walking to the car. And sure, they do drop pounds—often a lot in a short period of time. The trouble here, though, is twofold: for one, they end up losing a good deal of muscle tissue, which makes them appear stringy and shapeless; even worse, they depress their metabolism, ultimately leading to the dreaded rebound effect where all their previous weight is regained . . . and then some. Needless to say, this approach is seriously misguided.

Rest assured, if you don't exercise, you won't reshape your body. It's that simple. Only by combining exercise with a sensible nutritional program can you reap optimal results. Exercise truly *is* the elusive fountain of youth!

The Less Is More Philosophy

The good news is that you don't need to spend hours in the gym to achieve a terrific body. Far from it. Not only are marathon workouts unnecessary, but they can actually be counterproductive, suppressing your immune system and impairing progress. As you'll soon discover, it's the quality of training—not the quantity—that produces results. All that's required for my 28-Day Shapeover program is approximately three hours a week of exercise. That's right, three hours! In the case of exercise, less really can be more.

One of the biggest exercise-related complaints I hear from women is that they can't find the time to train. Perhaps you're in the same boat, constantly juggling your agenda, trying to fit a multitude of responsibilities into a limited amount of time. If this is a concern, you're in luck; my 28-Day Shapeover program is designed for maximum flexibility, allowing you to tailor it to your lifestyle, no matter how busy you might be. It is laid out as a six-day-a-week routine, alternating between a 30- to 40-minute weightlifting session one day and a 30-minute cardio session the next (with one day a week that is free from any strenuous exercise). This allows you ample opportunities to get in a quickie workout whenever time allows.

Perhaps, though, it's too taxing for you to work out six days a week? No problem. Simply combine the cardio and weight workouts into one session. In this case, you'll exercise three days per week, working out every other day for about an hour. You'll spend a little more time in a session when you opt for this approach, but training frequency is cut in half.

All things considered, it doesn't really matter which option you choose: both will generate the desired results. The most important thing is to make exercise a habit. Adherence is paramount. After all, what good is having the perfect routine if you don't follow it? Decide which option works best and then commit to it. If your schedule allows only brief workouts, then the first option would probably be the way to go; on the other hand, if fitting in a bigger block of time to exercise isn't a problem and you'd rather have more days off from training, then option two is the better bet. Either way, make sure that you adhere to a regimented schedule. Given the time-efficient nature of my program, there is no way to claim you can't fit a workout into your busy schedule.

The EPOC Advantage

One of the reasons my shapeover program is so effective is that it maximizes a phenomenon called excess postexercise oxygen consumption (EPOC). In a nutshell, EPOC is a measure of the calories that you burn *after* your workout is finished. Contrary to what you may have been led to believe, your metabolism remains elevated for a period of time following training. Moreover, there is an increased secretion of both growth hormone and noradrenaline—hormones that help to mobilize adipose stores, increasing the utilization of fat for fuel. All told, this results in both a greater total amount of calories expended as well as a greater amount of fat oxidation following training.

Here's the catch, though: EPOC is intensity dependent—the harder you train, the more calories you expend following training. I've harnessed this concept to create my unique program. You will train hard—probably a lot harder than you're used to training. But provided you're willing to put in the effort, you'll see—as so many other women have over the years—that the results are well worth it!

Lift to Lose

Although any type of exercise can be beneficial to losing body fat, resistance training (i.e., lifting weights) is by far the most important activity in the shapeover process. Not only does it help to tone your muscles (other exercise modalities have little if any effect in this regard), but it also plays an integral role in promoting fat loss. The reason has to do with the metabolic properties of muscle tissue. Muscle is, far and away, the most metabolically active tissue in your body. For each pound of muscle you carry, you burn up to an additional 50 calories a day. Better yet, you burn these calories on a continual basis, even when you're lying on the couch watching your favorite TV program! To put this in perspective, by gaining a mere five pounds of lean muscle, you'll burn an additional 1,750 calories a week, regardless of activity level. Assuming you keep food consumption constant, those five pounds of muscle will result in a net loss of about 25 pounds of fat in just one year's time!

What's more, resistance training promotes a significantly greater EPOC than cardio, with effects lasting for more than 38 hours! So even though you might not expend as much energy during exercise performance, weight training ultimately allows you to burn a greater amount of fat in total.

Given these facts, resistance training is at the core of my 28-Day Body Shapeover program. Let's now discuss the basics of the routine in detail.

Variety Is the Spice of Fitness

Variety is the spice of fitness. This is a motto I live by and one that I'm constantly preaching in my books and seminars, and to my private clients. And when it comes to resistance training, the importance of training variety cannot be overstated. Here's why: the human body is the most resourceful of all organisms and intuitively adapts to repetitive stress, including that from exercise. Accordingly, it becomes "immune" to exercises when they are performed over and over again. The longer you stay with the same routine, the less effective it becomes.

The key to continued progress is to interject constant variety into your routine. Doing so keeps your body "off-guard," never giving it the opportunity to get accustomed to a particular muscular stress. Your muscles are thereby forced to adjust to new stresses, ultimately fostering their ongoing development.

To take maximum advantage of the concept of variety, my 28-Day Body Shapeover regimen employs a technique called *nonlinear periodization*, where performance variables are constantly altered over the course of the month. You'll perform a different routine each time you work out, varying the exercises, reps, sets, and rest intervals from one week to the next. What's more, you'll utilize various specialized techniques designed to blast through training plateaus and shock your muscles into development. Not only will your workouts remain fresh and interesting, but in addition, you'll soon see your body change like you never thought possible.

Combine Exercises for Optimal Effect

With respect to exercise, the concept of variety needs to be expanded beyond simply performing an array of exercises; you also need to take into account how these movements interact with each other. Basic kinesiology dictates that certain exercises are complementary, working synergistically to produce optimal results. Unfortunately, even many fitness professionals do not fully comprehend this process and continue to train their clients in a haphazard fashion, stringing together a series of exercises without regard to how they mesh.

Muscles are made up of many thousands of tiny, threadlike fibers. In many cases, these fibers have different attachments that often run in different directions across the muscle. Thus, to fully develop a muscle, you must work all of the fibers within the muscle. The flat chest press, for instance, primarily works the middle and lower portions of the pectorals (sternoclavicular head). You can attain a good degree of chest development by using this exercise. However, by combining the flat chest press with an incline chest press, the upper fibers of the pectorals (clavicular head) will become much more active, resulting in a more symmetrical appearance. By adding in a fly movement, even more fibers are recruited, further improving results.

On the other hand, there would be little gained from performing both incline barbell presses and incline dumbbell presses in the same workout. These movements essentially target the same areas of the chest. Utilizing both of them in the same session would be superfluous and cause you to expend valuable energy reserves that could be put to better use.

In my shapeover regimen, you won't have to worry about deciding which exercises mesh best; I've done all the legwork for you. Each exercise has been specifically chosen to target different areas of the muscle complex you are working on that particular day. You'll enjoy a perfect workout every time you train, working the full spectrum of muscle fibers over the course of the program.

Split It Up

The composition of the resistance training routine is structured as a three-day *split routine*, where you train each muscle group once per week. A split routine allows you to blast a muscle group from multiple angles and then provides adequate time for muscular recovery. The following is the weekly split that will be employed:

- **Workout One:** Shoulders, biceps, triceps
- **Workout Two:** Quadriceps, hamstrings, calves
- **Workout Three:** Back, chest, abdominals

In order to facilitate optimal recovery, you will rest for at least 48 hours between resistance training sessions. This is the approximate length of time for protein synthesis to take place (the process by which your body repairs muscle tissue), and it ensures complete recuperation from the previous workout. So if you start the routine on Monday, then day two will fall on a Wednesday, and day three on a Friday (you can also do Tuesday, Thursday, Saturday, or Wednesday, Friday, Sun, etc.).

Raise Workout Intensity

Of all the tenets of exercise, none is more essential than intensity (i.e., how hard you work out). With respect to resistance training, intensity is dictated by the *overload principle*. Simply stated, this means that your muscles must be stressed beyond their physical capacity in order to develop.

By nature, the human body strives to maintain stability—a phenomenon called homeostasis. If your intensity of effort doesn't sufficiently tax your muscles and push them beyond what they are previously used to lifting, there won't be enough of a stimulus to force them from their homeostatic state. Only by progressively overloading your muscles will they be compelled to produce an adaptive response and develop beyond their normal potential.

A lack of intensity is the biggest downfall for most women in their quest for a better body; they simply don't train hard enough to effect change in their physiques. Many seem to feel that using light weights is the best way to tone up and thus they never provide enough of an impetus for their muscles to develop (I've actually seen trainees talking on the cell phone and reading magazines while doing exercises such as leg presses and biceps curls!). Needless to say, such an approach is destined to lead to substandard results.

In my 28-Day Shapeover program, you will train beyond your comfort zone, pushing yourself to complete each set. You won't think of weights as heavy or light. These are nebulous terms that have little practical meaning. A weight that is heavy for one person may be light for another. Rather, you'll choose a weight that is heavy enough so that the last few repetitions become difficult, if not impossible, to finish. Training in this fashion will provide stimulus for your muscles to develop to their fullest potential.

At least some of your sets should be taken to the point of momentary muscular failure—the point at which you are physically unable to perform another rep. For those not used to this approach, you will have to alter your mind-set to ensure that true failure is attained. It is human nature to seek pleasure and avoid pain. Pushing your body beyond the pain threshold is a daunting task. When a muscle is overloaded, lactic acid is produced, causing the burn in the muscle that ultimately leads to muscular fatigue. Although the natural temptation is to give into the burn, it is essential to push past this sensation. If you perform your desired number of repetitions and are still able to get several more, you have not sufficiently taxed the muscle and your results will be compromised. Make sure that your mind isn't giving up before your body. To achieve optimal results, you must disregard the pain threshold and completely fatigue your target muscles.

Where to Train

If possible, it's generally best to work out in a health club. A good fitness facility will have a vast selection of fitness equipment available for use and, as you'll soon learn, the more variety you can interject into your routine, the better. Barbells, dumbbells, machines, cables, plate-loaded equipment—there is simply no way for most people to have this type of variety in a home gym.

With that said, cost, convenience, and comfort are all valid reasons why you might prefer training at home. Given the importance of exercise adherence, you need to structure your training based on what works for you.

To satisfy all preferences, I have provided both gym-based and home-based routines for each session. If you should opt to go it at home, the following equipment will be needed:

- **Dumbbells:** Dumbbells are an essential component of any home gym. You probably will need a set of 2-, 3-, 5-, 8-, 10-, 12-, 15-, and 20-pound dumbbells. Depending on your strength levels, additional dumbbells might be necessary.

- **Ankle weights:** Ankle weights provide increased resistance for body-weight movements. Get ones that can accommodate 10-pound weight insertions. Depending on your strength level, a second set may be necessary.

- **Elastic strength bands:** Strength bands simulate cable exercise movements. Because they have a unique strength-curve, they are an excellent complement to free weight exercises.

- **Bench:** Although not an absolute necessity, it is advisable to buy an adjustable weight bench. This will allow you to train at an incline, affording the ability to vary your movements and hit your muscles from different angles. If you don't have the room for a bench, then you can use a Swiss ball as an alternative for many of the exercises—it's not as versatile as a good quality bench and has a downside in that it forces you to use lighter weights, but it will suffice for the intended purpose.

The Art of Cardio

By stating that resistance training is the most important activity you can perform, I do not mean to diminish the benefits of cardio (also known as *aerobic exercise*). Besides having a positive effect on your cardiovascular health, aerobic exercise also plays a significant role in body aesthetics. Here are some of the reasons you need to add a cardio component to your exercise routine:

- *Cardio expedites fat burning.* A single half-hour session of cardio, performed as outlined in my 28-Day Shapeover program, can burn hundreds of extra calories during the performance of the activity. Better yet, there is a boost in EPOC following cardiovascular training, prolonging fat-burning effects for up to several hours postworkout. What's more, your mitochondria (cellular furnaces where fat burning takes place) expand in size and number, and your aerobic enzymes (chemical messengers that accelerate the fat-burning process) increase in quantity. Over time, these factors allow your body to rely more on utilizing fat rather than glycogen (carbohydrate), for fuel, helping to sustain long-term weight management.

- *Cardio improves muscular endurance.* When you lift weights, your body converts glucose into the high-energy compound ATP (through a process called glycolysis) to fuel exercise performance. During this conversion process, lactic acid is produced and rapidly accumulates in your muscles as you train. When lactic acid builds up past a certain point, you experience an intense burning sensation in your muscles. Ultimately, the burn becomes so strong that it impedes your ability to achieve a muscular contraction; at that point, you simply cannot continue to train. However, by increasing aerobic capacity, your cardiovascular system becomes more efficient at delivering oxygen to your working muscles. This helps to increase your lactate threshold—the point at which there is more lactic acid in your body than can be metabolized—and thereby delays the onset of lactic acid buildup. The end result is a greater capacity to train at a high level of intensity.

- *Cardio enhances muscular recuperation.* Aerobic exercise helps to expand your network of capillaries—the tiny blood vessels that allow nutrients such as protein and carbohydrate to be absorbed into body tissues. The more capillaries that you have, the more efficient your body becomes in utilizing these nutrients for muscular repair. Capillaries also help to clear waste products, particularly carbon dioxide, from the food-burning process, further enhancing the efficiency of your nutrient-delivery system. This accelerates the rate at which your muscles are able to get the resources needed for recuperation, helping to improve workouts and speed recovery.

There are two basic factors that influence the fat-burning effects of cardio: duration (how long you train) and intensity (how hard you train). For any given level of calories burned, these factors have an inverse relationship: if you train harder, then you don't have to train as long; if you train longer, then you don't have to train as hard.

However, both research and experience have shown that a specific type of cardio known as *interval training* provides significant benefits over steady state exercise. For one, interval training is extremely time efficient, allowing you to complete a workout in about half the time of traditional cardio protocols. For another, interval training is more effective at burning fat than comparable steady state exercise. In large part, this is because of an increased effect on EPOC, in which fat burning is prolonged well after you finish the activity.

In my 28-Day Shapeover program, you will perform "high-energy" intervals. In essence, this involves combining high-intensity and low-intensity intervals in a way that maximizes fat burning. I've structured the routines so they have minimal redundancy, varying in intensity, duration, and mode. You'll always be challenged, never bored.

During the high-intensity intervals, you will train for one minute at a level that exceeds your lactate threshold. This will be followed by a lower-intensity interval of between one and four minutes, where your body has a chance to clear lactic acid from the blood and replenish oxygen stores. The cycle will be repeated multiple times over the course of the cardio workout, allowing you to burn in excess of 300 calories in just thirty minutes.

You will monitor the intensity of intervals using a concept called a *rating of perceived exertion* (RPE). Simply stated, RPE is a measure of how hard you feel like you are exercising. It takes into account the physical sensations you experience during exercise, including increases in heart rate, breathing rate, sweating, and muscle fatigue. In this book, RPE is rated using an incremental scale ranging from one to ten, with one representing a lack of exertion and ten representing maximum possible exertion. For example, a three would indicate a level of exertion that is fairly easy, while an eight would indicate a level of exertion that is very demanding.

As opposed to other forms of cardio you might be used to performing, high-energy interval training is quite physically demanding. Depending on your level of aerobic fitness, you may have trouble getting through an entire workout at the suggested RPE levels. If this is the case, don't worry; simply decrease RPE on the higher-intensity intervals to a level more consistent with your abilities. As time goes by and you achieve greater aerobic fitness, try to gradually increase the RPEs until you are training at the prescribed intensity. Aerobic fitness tends to improve at a rapid rate and it shouldn't be long before you're able to proceed at the suggested levels of intensity.

Probably the question most often asked about cardio is, "What aerobic activity burns the most calories?" In truth, there is no "best" cardiovascular exercise. It all comes down to duration and intensity. If you perform two different activities with a similar duration and intensity, then you will achieve similar results in terms of calories burned. (There will be some individual variances based on genetic factors, but their overall effect is relatively minor.)

Your best approach is to choose exercises that you like doing. If you enjoy an activity, you'll be more likely to stick with it over the long haul. That said, I would encourage you to try to keep an open mind and experiment with as many different activities as possible; sometimes you'll enjoy an exercise more as time goes on. As with resistance training, variety is an important part of cardiovascular exercise. As previously noted, the human body readily adjusts to an external stimulus by becoming more proficient. Therefore, when the same exercise is used repeatedly, adaptation takes place, ultimately leading to diminished returns.

With respect to cardio, variety is referred to as *cross-training*. Cross-training can be accomplished by performing as few as two different activities (although the more, the better) and alternating them from one workout to the next. Not only does this keep your body off-guard, but it also helps to reduce the likelihood of a training-related injury. Since each modality uses different muscles in exercise performance, your bones, muscles, and joints aren't subjected to continual impact. There is less wear and tear on your body, saving your musculoskeletal system from overuse.

For the cardio component of my shapeover program, I have suggested using the treadmill, stair climber, and stationary bike. These modalities have the advantage of being widely available for home or gym use; they can be performed regardless of weather conditions; and they have the capability to adjust intensity levels to facilitate performance of cardio intervals. That said, don't feel locked into these exercises. As I mentioned previously, it's important to choose modalities you enjoy. Virtually any activity can be adapted to interval training, and I've employed outdoor running, jumping rope, rowing, elliptical training, and a host of other modalities with my private clients.

Stay Flexible

All too often, stretching tends to be the forgotten fitness component. Not only does flexibility have positive effects on your posture and mobility, but it also can help to reduce the risk of a joint-related injury. And remember, if you're injured, you can't train. . . and if you can't train, you can't tone up your body!

Contrary to popular belief, resistance training in itself actually helps to improve flexibility. Provided that you train as directed, your joints will be taken through their full stretch capacity, thereby facilitating better range of motion. This has been proven in research: studies have consistently shown that those who lift weights are, on average, more limber than those who don't.

But resistance training alone isn't enough to optimize flexibility. In order to achieve this goal, my 28-Day Shapeover program incorporates a technique called *selective muscular stretching* into the workouts. This involves stretching the muscle trained in between resistance training sets. As soon as you finish a set, you will initiate the stretch and hold it throughout your rest period.

Not only is selective muscular stretching a time-efficient way to enhance flexibility, it also helps to improve muscular recovery between sets. It does this by helping to flush lactic acid from your muscles. If you recall, lactic acid is a by-product of ATP—the primary source of energy used to fuel your muscles during anaerobic exercise. By restoring blood flow to your working muscles, selective muscular stretching rapidly regenerates your muscular capacity, allowing you to come back strong for your next set.

The following are descriptions and illustrations of the stretches you will use in the course of your routine.

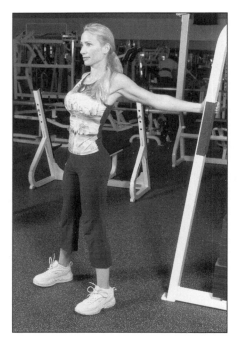

Chest Stretch

From a standing position, grasp a stationary object (such as a pole or exercise machine) with your right hand. Your arm should be straight and roughly parallel to the ground. Slowly turn away from the object, allowing your arm to go as far behind your body as comfortably possible. Hold this position for the desired time then repeat the process with your left arm.

Shoulder Stretch

From a standing position, grasp your right wrist or elbow with your left hand. Without turning your body, slowly pull your right arm across your torso as far as comfortably possible. Hold this position for the desired time then repeat the process with your left arm.

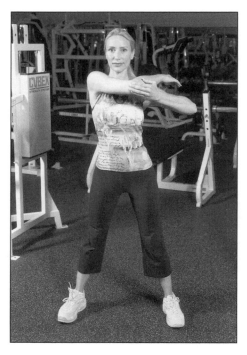

Upper Back Stretch

From a standing position, grasp a stationary object (such as a pole or exercise machine) with both hands. Bend your knees and sit back so that your arms are fully extended and supporting your weight. Shift your weight to the right to isolate the right portion of your lat muscle. Hold this position for the desired time and then shift your weight to the left.

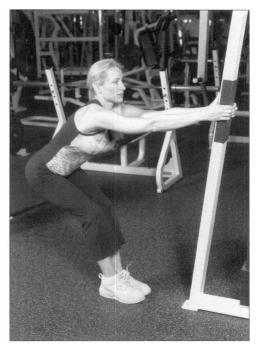

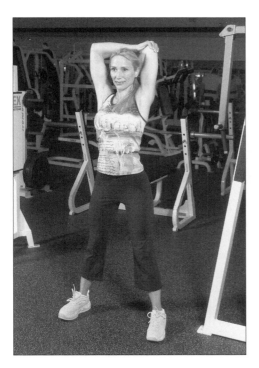

Triceps Stretch

From a standing position, raise your right arm over your head. Bend your elbow so that your right hand is behind your head. With your left hand, grasp your right wrist or elbow and pull it back as far as comfortably possible, pointing your right elbow toward the ceiling. Hold this position for the desired time then repeat the process with your left arm.

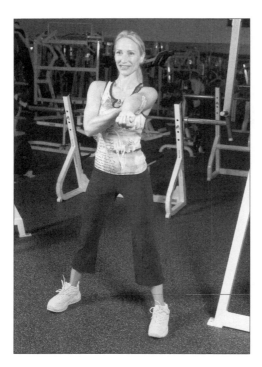

Biceps Stretch

From a standing position, extend your right arm forward with your palm facing up. Place your left palm underneath your right elbow. Slowly straighten your right arm as much as comfortably possible, pressing your elbow down into your left hand. Hold this position for the desired time then repeat the process with your left arm.

Glute/Hamstring Stretch

Sit on the floor with your legs straight and slowly bend forward. Allow your hands to travel down along the line of your body as far as comfortably possible. When you feel an intense stretch in your hamstrings, grab onto your legs and hold this position for the desired time.

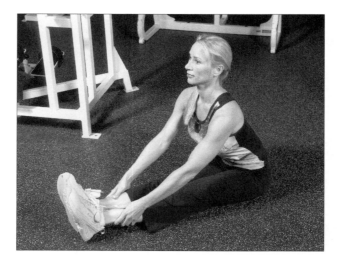

Quadriceps Stretch

From a standing position, grasp a stationary object (such as a pole or exercise machine) with your right hand. Bend your left knee and bring your left foot toward your butt. Grasp your left ankle or foot with your left hand and slowly lift your foot as high as comfortably possible. Hold this position for the desired time then repeat the process with your right leg.

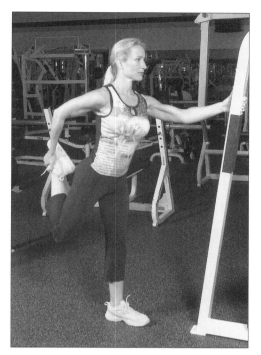

Calf Stretch

From a standing position, grasp a stationary object (such as a pole or exercise machine) with both hands. Bend your right knee and bring your left leg behind your body as far as you can while keeping your feet flat on the floor. Slowly lean forward without lifting your left heel. Hold this position for the desired time then repeat the process with your right leg.

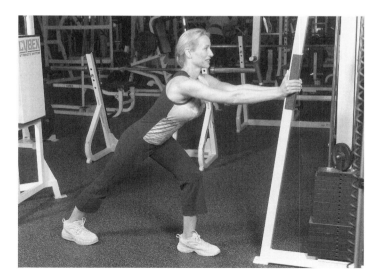

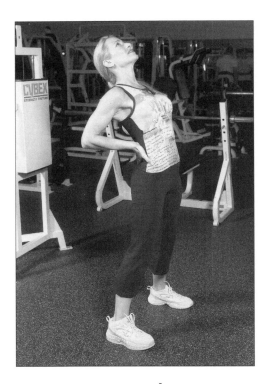

Ab Stretch

From a standing position, place your hands on your sides and slowly lean back as far as comfortably possible. For added effect and to enhance the stretch on the oblique muscles, lean to your left and then to your right while performing this stretch.

Shapeover Nutrition

When it comes to shaping over your body, nutrition and exercise go hand in hand; it's the proverbial 50/50 proposition. In addition to playing a role in whether you gain or lose body fat, what you eat also fuels exercise performance and promotes the development of lean muscle tissue. If you don't supply your body with the proper nutrients, you'll seriously compromise your workouts and results will suffer (or cease to exist!).

The nutritional component of my shapeover program is similar to the type of regimen I prescribe for fitness and figure competitors who are training for competition. It provides you with the right combination of the right amounts of the right foods, allowing you to lose weight safely and efficiently, reducing fat without cannibalizing muscle tissue. Ultimately, you'll attain a super-lean physique that is both firm and shapely.

As with the exercise program, my aim here is to make the diet as user friendly as possible. As such, each meal is laid out in menu-style fashion, down to the exact portion size. There is no guesswork; all you have to do is eat!

Unlike other diets, you will eat from all three major food groups, with balanced portions of carbs, protein, and fat included in each daily menu. Contrary to what you may have heard from so-called nutritional gurus, all of these nutrients have a place in a balanced meal plan and, when properly integrated into a regimen, help to power your body during intense exercise and stoke your internal furnace.

I've taken great care to provide a variety of different foods each day, ensuring that you'll never get tired of the diet. Like exercise, adherence is paramount to an effective nutritional regimen. Boredom quickly leads to noncompliance, and often precipitates uncontrolled binge eating. Given the diverse selection here, that won't happen with this program.

Instead of the traditional "three squares" a day, you'll eat five daily meals—breakfast, lunch, and dinner, plus two snack meals. As you'll come to learn, frequent feedings are an important component in attaining a lean, hard physique, helping to rev up your metabolism and keep hunger at bay. It's one of the surefire ways to turn your body into a fat-burning machine.

Finally, you'll eat the bulk of your starchy carbs early in the day, when they can be best used to fuel your daily activities. If carbs are not used immediately for energy, they have two possible fates; they're either stored as glycogen in your liver and muscles, or are indirectly (or in some cases directly) converted into fatty acids and stored as body fat. Because activity levels usually are lowest during the evening hours, you'll stick with protein and fibrous vegetables at this time, reducing the potential for unwanted fat storage.

The timing of carb consumption can have an effect on your body's response to insulin. Insulin sensitivity tends to be highest in the morning, meaning your body is better able to assimilate carbs at this time. As the day wears on, insulin sensitivity gradually diminishes, and, by evening, it's at its lowest point. Hence, carbs eaten at night evoke a greater insulin response, fueling the processes that facilitate fat storage and suppress fat burning. And there's even a carryover effect to the next day. Eating a carbohydrate rich dinner tends to increase the insulin response of the following morning's meal. So, not only are insulin levels elevated after dinner, but they remain that way through breakfast, too. By eating your starches early, you'll take maximum advantage of your body's diurnal clock, creating an environment favorable to burning fat.

Now it is time to begin 28 days of hard work, determination, and intense workouts, aiming at that one goal: to transform your body. Let's get started!

Week One

2

Congratulations—you're ready to begin the 28-Day Shapeover program! Just carrying through with your commitment to exercise and eating right is more than half the battle when it comes to getting into shape. If you adhere to the program as directed, you will see terrific results, guaranteed. So put on your gym clothes, lace up your sneakers, and get ready to work up a sweat!

The training protocol for Week One focuses on maximizing muscular development. Now before you start thinking that you're going to end up looking like one of those hulking female bodybuilders you've seen in magazines, think again. It would be physiologically impossible to bulk up in a week's time—or a even a month's, for that matter. This is the last thing you need to worry about.

In truth, it's extremely difficult for the vast majority of women to develop large muscles, period—even if they make a concerted effort over time. The main reason: a lack of testosterone. Testosterone is a hormone that's secreted by the testes (in males) and, to a lesser extent, by the ovaries (in females). It has two main functions: First, testosterone is *androgenic* (i.e., masculinizing); it promotes male-oriented characteristics such as the growth of facial and body hair, male-pattern baldness, and deepening of the voice. Second, testosterone is *anabolic* (building); through a complex process, it interacts at the cellular level with muscle tissue to increase protein synthesis—the primary stimulus for initiating muscular growth. Hence, there is a direct relationship between testosterone and muscle mass: the more testosterone you secrete, the greater your propensity to pack on muscle.

On average, women produce only about one-tenth the amount of testosterone as their male counterparts; this is nature's way of preserving femininity. As a result, it's difficult for women to add a significant amount of muscular bulk to their frame. Without an anabolic stimulus, muscle tissue simply has no impetus to hypertrophy (grow larger) and muscular growth remains modest, even at advanced levels of training.

If you follow the protocol as described, you should be able to add about a half-pound to a pound of lean muscle over the course of the week. The addition of shapely muscle will not only improve your body lines, but will also increase your metabolism and thus expedite the loss of body fat (remember, each pound of added muscle burns up to 50 extra calories a day at rest!).

Let's go over the exercise protocol for Week One in detail.

Resistance Training Protocol

Sets   You will perform two to four sets of each exercise. The sets will be executed in a straight fashion, meaning you'll do a set, stretch for the prescribed amount of time, do another set, stretch, and so on. You'll finish all sets for a particular exercise before moving on to the next exercise.

For example, in the Day 1 workout, you'll begin by performing a shoulder press. After executing the specified number of repetitions, you'll stretch the target muscle group, perform another set of shoulder presses, stretch again, and then perform a final set of shoulder presses. You'll then move to your next exercise and proceed in a similar manner for the rest of the workout.

Repetitions   You will employ a moderate repetition scheme, aiming for 8 to 10 reps per set. A moderate rep scheme is ideal for inducing muscle hypertrophy. Here's why:

- **Muscle Fiber Activation:** Clearly, maximal growth can only be achieved by activating the full spectrum of muscle fibers. A moderate rep scheme accomplishes this better than either a very low rep scheme or a very high rep scheme. Both slow-twitch and fast-twitch muscle fibers are brought into play, and the time under tension is long enough to work these muscles to their fullest potential. (See the sidebar about muscle fibers for a detailed explanation of this phenomenon.)

- **Hormonal Excitation:** Moderate reps have been shown to maximize the release of various hormones, including testosterone and growth hormone. This process is facilitated by the accrual of lactic acid. Although the exact mechanism is unclear, it has been shown that lactate promotes hormonal excitation, which then acts on the muscle cell to induce growth.

- **Cellular Hydration:** Moderate rep training causes a distinct muscular "pump" in which your muscles engorge with blood. This not only provides a temporary fullness to your muscles, but also increases hydration within the muscle cells. Numerous studies have demonstrated that a hydrated cell stimulates protein synthesis and inhibits proteolysis (protein breakdown). In this way, muscles are provided with the raw materials to lay down new contractile proteins—the primary basis for muscle growth.

In accordance with the overload principle, the weight you choose must be heavy enough so that the last few reps of the set are difficult, if not impossible, to complete. If you're not struggling on the last few reps, the weight is too light. Alternatively, if you are not able to execute at least eight full reps, the weight is too heavy. With a little experimentation, you'll soon have a handle on exactly how much weight you should use for each exercise.

The only exception to the moderate rep protocol is the seated calf raise. This exercise targets the soleus muscle, which is comprised almost predominantly of slow-twitch muscle fibers and thus responds best to high rep training. Thus, you'll perform 15 to 20 reps for seated calf raises.

Understanding Muscle Fibers

Muscles are comprised of thousands of tiny, threadlike fibers. There are two basic types of muscle fibers: type I and type II, and each plays different roles in muscle function.

Type I fibers are called slow-twitch fibers. They are endurance oriented and have only a limited ability to increase in size. These fibers get much of their energy by burning fat for fuel, contracting very slowly but having the ability to endure extended periods of activity.

Type II fibers are called fast-twitch fibers. These fibers are strength-related; they contract rapidly but are quick to fatigue. Most of their energy is derived by burning glucose, rather than fat, as a fuel source, and they have the greatest potential for hypertrophy (i.e., growth).

Almost any type of resistance training uses a combination of both type I and type II fibers. However, the repetition range that you employ influences the activation of these fibers. Here's why: Fibers are recruited according to the *size principle*. Smaller, type I fibers are activated first, corresponding to lighter weight, higher rep training. As heavier weights are used, larger, type II fibers are progressively brought into play until all the available fibers have been recruited. This is the reason that higher rep training does not significantly increase muscular size: the weights used just aren't heavy enough to fully stimulate type II fibers—the ones with the greatest potential for growth.

Rest Intervals   You will rest between 60 to 90 seconds between sets. Given the moderate repetition range (and corresponding heavier weight load), your muscles will need a little longer to recuperate than with a higher rep/lighter load scheme. Resting 60 to 90 seconds has proven to be sufficient so that you can come back strong on successive sets while keeping your anabolic levels high.

During the rest period, you will employ a technique known as *selective muscular stretching*. The concept is simple: as soon as a set is completed, you'll immediately stretch the muscle being trained. Try to hold each stretch for the entire rest interval and then proceed directly to your next set (see chapter 1 for descriptions and illustrations of the appropriate stretches).

When you stretch, go only to the point where you feel tension in the muscle—not to where you experience unbearable pain. If you stretch too far, your body sends a neural impulse to the overstretched muscle (called the *stretch reflex*), causing it to contract. This reflex actually tightens the muscle, creating the opposite effect of what you are trying to accomplish. By stretching slowly, you can ease into a comfortable zone, taking your body to the edge without going over. Finally, make sure to keep yourself loose and relaxed during the stretch, breathing in a slow, rhythmic fashion.

Cardio Protocol

The cardio component during Week One will aid in expediting fat loss while you're gaining muscle. This week's routine is designed to introduce you to high-energy interval training. As previously noted, you will perform staggered intervals, varying between low-intensity and high-intensity training. The intervals will follow a "bell-shaped" curve. You will start out with a warm-up and then proceed to intervals going from 4:1 down to 2:1 and then back up to 4:1, before finishing with a cool-down.

I have suggested the treadmill, stationary bike, and stair climber as the modalities of choice, but feel free to substitute alternative exercises at your discretion. If possible, try to cross-train using at least two different movements from session to session to allow for sufficient variety. Also, please note that there are many different makes and models of treadmills, stationary bikes, and stair climbers. Take some time to acclimate yourself to the features of your selected unit, and, if possible, talk with a gym employee or read the owner's manual so you can best take advantage of what the machine has to offer.

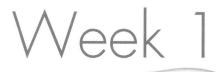

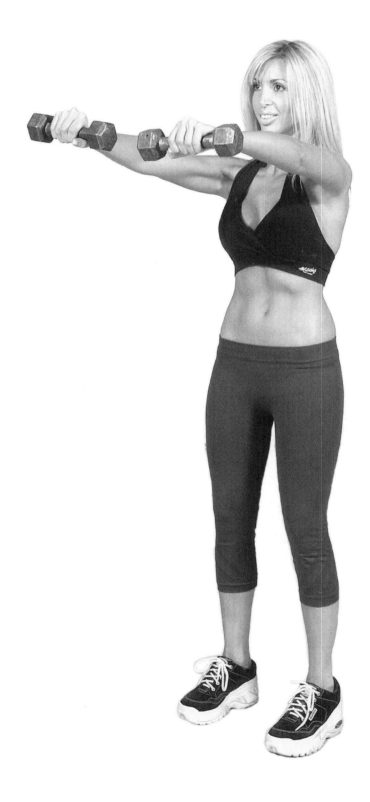

Resistance and Cardio Workouts

Day 1

Workout

Today will be a resistance workout. You'll train shoulders, biceps, and triceps. Remember to selectively stretch the muscle group you are training between sets. Stretches for shoulders, triceps, and biceps are shown on pages 10, 11, and 12, respectively.

Gym	Sets	Reps	Home
Dumbbell Shoulder Press 113	4	8 to 10	Dumbbell Shoulder Press 113
Cable Rope Upright Row 115	3	8 to 10	Dumbbell Upright Row 114
Kneeling Cable Bent Lateral Raise 118	3	8 to 10	Dumbbell Bent Lateral Raise 119
One-Arm Cable Curl 129	3	8 to 10	One-Arm Strength Band Curl 131
Barbell Drag Curl 124	2	8 to 10	Dumbbell Drag Curl 125
Dumbbell Concentration Curl 132	2	8 to 10	Dumbbell Concentration Curl 132

Gym	Sets	Reps	Home
Dumbbell Triceps Kickback 137	3	8 to 10	Dumbbell Triceps Kickback 137
One-Arm Dumbbell Overhead Triceps Extension 143	3	8 to 10	One-Arm Dumbbell Overhead Triceps Extension 143
One-Arm Cable Reverse Pressdown 139	2	8 to 10	One-Arm Strength Band Reverse Pressdown 140

Menu

Meal One

- 1/2 cup oatmeal
- 1 scoop whey protein powder
- Coffee or tea

Meal Two

- Strawberry smoothie (containing 1 cup strawberries, 1 scoop whey protein powder, 1 tablespoon flax oil, and crushed ice)

Meal Three

- 6 ounces grilled chicken breast
- Large salad (containing romaine lettuce, green pepper, carrot, tomato, balsamic vinegar, and 1 tablespoon olive oil)

Meal Four

- 1 medium pear

Meal Five

- 6 ounces flounder
- 12 ounces grilled yellow squash

Day 2

Workout

Today will be a cardio workout. You'll be performing your training on the treadmill. I have provided target RPE intervals along with corresponding suggestions for enhancing intensity by varying the angle of incline and stride pace.

Minutes	RPE	Notes
3	3	Warm up at low intensity. No incline.
4	5	Slightly increase stride pace. No incline.
1	7	Increase stride pace. Increase the incline .5% every 30 seconds.
3	5	Decrease stride pace. Maintain current incline.
1	8	Increase stride pace. Increase the incline .5% every 30 seconds.
2	5	Decrease stride pace. Maintain current incline.
1	9	Increase stride pace. Increase the incline .5% every 30 seconds.
2	5	Decrease stride pace. Decrease the incline .5% every 30 seconds.
1	9	Increase stride pace. Maintain current incline.
3	5	Decrease stride pace. Decrease the incline .5% every 30 seconds.
1	8	Increase stride pace. Maintain current incline.
4	5	Decrease stride pace. Decrease the incline .5% every 30 seconds.
1	7	Increase stride pace. Maintain current incline.
3	3	Cool down at low intensity. No incline.

Day 2

Menu

Meal One

- 2 slices multigrain bread
- Mushroom omelet (containing 6 egg whites and 1 large portabella mushroom)
- 1 tablespoon flaxseed oil
- Coffee or tea

Meal Two

- 1 ounce raw, unsalted peanuts

Meal Three

- Turkey sandwich (containing 4 ounces sliced turkey breast on seven-grain bread)
- Large salad (containing romaine lettuce, green pepper, carrot, tomato, onion, balsamic vinegar, and 1 tablespoon olive oil)

Meal Four

- 1 cup raspberries

Meal Five

- 6 ounces broiled bay scallops
- 12 ounces spinach

Day 3

Workout

Today will be a resistance workout. You'll be training thighs (quadriceps), butt (glutes), and calves. Remember to selectively stretch the muscle group you are training between sets. Stretches for glutes/hamstrings, quadriceps, and calves are shown on pages 12, 13, and 13, respectively.

Gym		Sets	Reps	Home	
Barbell Squat	150	4	8 to 10	Dumbbell Squat	152
One-Legged Machine Leg Extension	151	3	8 to 10	One-Legged Weighted Leg Extension	153
Dumbbell Side Lunge	152	3	8 to 10	Dumbbell Side Lunge	152
Dumbbell Stiff Legged Deadlift	162	3	8 to 10	Dumbbell Stiff Legged Deadlift	162
One-Legged Machine Lying Leg Curl	166	3	8 to 10	One-Legged Weighted Lying Leg Curl	169
Cable Standing Abductor Raise	171	2	8 to 10	Weighted Standing Abductor Raise	172

Day 3

Gym		Sets	Reps	Home	
Machine Standing Calf Raise	176	3	8 to 10	Dumbbell Standing Calf Raise	178
One-Legged Machine Seated Calf Raise	177	3	15 to 20	One-Legged Dumbbell Seated Calf Raise	178

Menu

Meal One

- 1 cup Kashi cereal
- 4 ounces 1% milk

Meal Two

- Banana smoothie (containing 1 large banana, 1 scoop whey protein powder, 1 tablespoon flaxseed oil, and crushed ice)

Meal Three

- 6 ounces Cornish game hen breast
- Large salad (containing romaine lettuce, green pepper, carrot, tomato, balsamic vinegar, and 1 tablespoon olive oil)

Meal Four

- 1 medium peach

Meal Five

- 6 ounces orange roughy
- 12 ounces stir-fried vegetable medley

Day 4

Workout

Today will be a cardio workout. You'll be performing your training on the stationary bike. I have provided target RPE intervals along with corresponding suggestions for enhancing intensity by varying the resistance and/or pedal speed.

Minutes	RPE	Notes
3	3	Warm up at low intensity.
4	5	Slightly increase resistance and/or pedal speed.
1	7	Increase resistance and/or pedal speed.
3	5	Decrease resistance and/or pedal speed.
1	8	Increase resistance and/or pedal speed.
2	5	Decrease resistance and/or pedal speed.
1	9	Increase resistance and/or pedal speed.
2	5	Decrease resistance and/or pedal speed.
1	9	Increase resistance and/or pedal speed.
3	5	Decrease resistance and/or pedal speed.
1	8	Increase resistance and/or pedal speed.
4	5	Decrease resistance and/or pedal speed.
1	7	Increase resistance and/or pedal speed.
3	3	Cool down at low intensity.

Menu

Meal One

- 2 slices multigrain bread
- Vegetable omelet (containing 6 egg whites and chopped green pepper, red bell pepper, spinach, and onion)
- 1 tablespoon flaxseed oil
- Coffee or tea

Meal Two

- 1 medium apple

Meal Three

- Chicken salad (containing 6 ounces of grilled chicken, mixed greens, and 1 tablespoon olive oil)
- 1 medium sweet potato

Meal Four

- 1 ounce raw, unsalted Brazil nuts

Meal Five

- 4 ounces broiled shrimp
- 12 ounces asparagus

Day 5

Workout

Today will be a resistance workout. You'll be training chest, back, and abdominals. Remember to selectively stretch the muscle group you are training between sets. Stretches for chest, back, and abdominals are on pages 10, 11, and 14, respectively.

Gym		Sets	Reps	Home	
Barbell Incline Press	186	4	8 to 10	Dumbbell Incline Press	188
Dumbbell Flat Press	187	3	8 to 10	Dumbbell Flat Press	187
Dumbbell Incline Fly	187	3	8 to 10	Dumbbell Incline Fly	187
Reverse Lat Pulldown	204	4	8 to 10	Strength Band Reverse Lat Pulldown	206
One-Arm Dumbbell Row	196	3	8 to 10	One-Arm Dumbbell Row	196
Cable Lying Pullover	200	3	8 to 10	Strength Band Lying Pullover	203

Day 5

Gym	Sets	Reps	Home
Twisting Crunch	3	8 to 10	Twisting Crunch
211			211
Hanging Knee Raise	3	8 to 10	Hanging Knee Raise
212			212

Menu

Meal One

- 6 ounces 1% cottage cheese
- 2 slices multigrain bread
- Coffee or tea

Meal Two

- 1 ounce raw, unsalted almonds

Meal Three

- Chickpea salad (containing 8 ounces chickpeas, romaine lettuce, green pepper, carrot, tomato, onion, balsamic vinegar, and 1 tablespoon olive oil)

Meal Four

- Blueberry smoothie (containing 1 cup blueberries, 1 scoop whey protein powder, 1 tablespoon flaxseed oil, and crushed ice)

Meal Five

- 6 ounces sea bass
- 12 ounces green beans

Day 6

Workout

Today will be a cardio workout. You'll be performing your training on the stair climber. I have provided target RPE intervals along with corresponding suggestions for enhancing intensity by varying the resistance and/or step speed.

Minutes	RPE	Notes
3	3	Warm up at low intensity.
4	5	Slightly increase resistance and/or step speed.
1	7	Increase resistance and/or step speed.
3	5	Decrease resistance and/or step speed.
1	8	Increase resistance and/or step speed.
2	5	Decrease resistance and/or step speed.
1	9	Increase resistance and/or step speed.
2	5	Decrease resistance and/or step speed.
1	9	Increase resistance and/or step speed.
3	5	Decrease resistance and/or step speed.
1	8	Increase resistance and/or step speed.
4	5	Decrease resistance and/or step speed.
1	7	Increase resistance and/or step speed.
3	3	Cool down at low intensity.

Day 6

Menu

Meal One

- 1 cup cream of wheat
- 1 tablespoon flaxseed oil
- 1 scoop whey protein powder
- Coffee or tea

Meal Two

- 1 medium peach

Meal Three

- 4 ounces seared tuna steak
- 1/2 cup brown rice

Meal Four

- 1 cup plain yogurt

Meal Five

- 4 ounces sirloin steak
- 12 ounces mixed green vegetables
- 1 tablespoon olive oil

Day 7

Workout

Today is an off-day from training—a day to allow your body to recuperate from the intense training that you've done the rest of the week. Try to avoid any strenuous activities. If desired, you can do some light cardio such as walking. Most important—enjoy yourself!

Menu

Meal One

- 1/2 cup multigrain cereal
- 1 scoop whey protein powder
- 1 tablespoon flaxseed oil
- Coffee or tea

Meal Two

- 1 ounce raw, unsalted pecans

Meal Three

- Roast beef sandwich (containing 4 ounces extra-lean roast beef on multigrain bread)
- Large salad (containing romaine lettuce, green pepper, carrot, tomato, onion, balsamic vinegar, and 1 tablespoon olive oil)

Meal Four

- 3 fresh apricots

Meal Five

- 6 ounces broiled seafood mix (clams, oysters, calamari, shrimp, and scallops)
- 12 ounces zucchini

3

Week Two

You are into Week Two of the 28-Day Shapeover program and should be acclimated to the intense nature of the routine. We're now going to mix things up and shift our focus to the development of lean muscle tone and muscular endurance. By using an altered repetition/rest interval scheme as well as the addition of some specialized training techniques, you'll simultaneously hone sleek muscle while initiating a heightened fat-burning effect throughout your workout.

Let's go over the protocol for Week Two in detail.

Resistance Training Protocol

Sets You will perform two or three sets of each exercise. Some sets will be performed straight while others will employ the use of supersets. A *superset* is two exercises performed consecutively, with no rest between them. Supersets increase workout intensity and, because of the limited rest intervals, heighten fat burning to an even greater degree. They also are extremely time efficient, allowing you to cut your workout time in half. Since a muscle begins to recuperate within several seconds after the completion of a set, you should attempt to move from one exercise to the other in an expeditious fashion during supersetted movements.

Supersets will be performed for those muscle groups that have an agonist/antagonist relationship. Agonist/antagonist muscles are opposing muscle groups where one muscle contracts while the other relaxes. The quadriceps/hamstrings, back/chest, and triceps/biceps all possess this yin-yang relationship. For example, when the biceps (agonist) are trained, the triceps (antagonist) act as stabilizers. Conversely, when the triceps are trained, they become the agonist, while the biceps play the role of the antagonist. The beauty of performing agonist/antagonist supersets (as opposed to other superset combinations) is that it allows you to generate a more forceful contraction on the second exercise in the series.

Repetitions　　You will employ a high repetition scheme, aiming for 15 to 20 reps per set. This will heighten local muscular endurance and improve the quality of muscle tissue (i.e., muscle tone) without promoting significant gains in muscle mass. If you remember, during a high rep set, the weights used aren't heavy enough to innervate the highest-threshold motor units. These motor units control the fast-twitch type II fibers—the ones that have the greatest potential for growth. Instead, the majority of work is accomplished by slow-twitch type I fibers, which are fatigue-resistant but have a limited ability to hypertrophy. The net effect is a hard, sleek muscle that can endure lengthy bouts of exercise.

Remember though: just because you'll be using lighter weights doesn't mean you won't be training hard. You still need to make sure that the last few reps of the set are difficult, if not impossible, to complete. If you're not struggling on the last few reps, increase the amount of weight so that the sets challenge your muscles. On the other hand, if you can't finish a minimum of 15 reps in a set, decrease the amount of weight accordingly. Staying within the target range will ensure optimal results.

Rest Intervals　　You will keep your rest intervals to a minimum, taking no more than 30 seconds between sets. As a rule, training should commence before you can fully catch your breath. This will create a distinct aerobic effect, keeping your heart rate elevated throughout the session. This results in a substantial increase in caloric expenditure, ultimately helping to elevate metabolism and reduce body fat.

For the straight sets, you'll perform a set, rest for 30 seconds, perform another set, rest for 30 seconds, and so on. For the supersets, you'll perform the first exercise, immediately perform the second exercise, rest for 30 seconds, and repeat.

During the rest interval, you will employ selective muscular stretching, stretching the muscle that is being worked. For the supersets, you'll stretch both the agonist and antagonist muscle groups, spending the first half of the rest period on the agonist and the second half on the antagonist.

Cardio Protocol

Now that you're somewhat acclimated to the program, the cardio protocol for Week Two will jack the intensity up a notch. This is accomplished both by having shorter low-intensity intervals and a higher absolute RPE (up to 9 on the RPE scale). Because intensity (along with duration) dictates caloric cost, you'll jack up the amount of fat burned during the session. Moreover, this will have a positive effect on EPOC, helping to elevate your metabolism long after the completion of the routine.

You'll start with a warm-up and then the intervals will quickly diminish from a ratio of 3:1 down to 1:1. Also, on your higher-intensity intervals, your rating of perceived exertion should escalate up to a 9 on the RPE scale. You'll end with a mild cool-down. If the new routine proves to be too much to handle, simply go back to the cardio protocol outlined in Week One. With persistence, you'll soon be able to pick up the pace.

I have suggested the treadmill, stair climber, and stationary bike as the modalities of choice. As always, feel free to substitute alternative exercises at your discretion but try to cross-train using at least two different movements, if possible.

Understanding Muscular Soreness

Given how hard you've been training, it's possible that your muscles are quite sore after each workout, perhaps remaining that way for several days postexercise. If so, there are some things you should know about this condition, generally referred to as delayed-onset muscle soreness (DOMS).

Contrary to popular belief, DOMS is totally unrelated to a buildup of lactic acid. Lactate is rapidly cleared from muscles following a workout. Within an hour or two postexercise, it is either completely oxidized or taken up (via the Cori cycle) and utilized for glycogen resynthesis. Since DOMS doesn't occur until at least 24 hours after a training session, it therefore follows that lactic acid cannot play a part in its cause.

Although the exact mechanisms are not fully understood, current theory suggests that DOMS is actually a product of damage to muscle tissue. It is fundamentally caused by eccentric exercise, where muscles are lengthening under extreme tension. Here is the proposed model: During eccentric activity, the contractile elements (actin and myosin) of working muscles exert a "braking" action in order to resist the forces of gravity. This produces small microtears in both the contractile elements and surface membrane (sarcolemma) of the associated muscle fibers. These microtears allow calcium to escape from the muscles, disrupting their intra-cellular balance and causing further injury to the fibers. Various proteins (such as neutrophils and macrophages) then interact with the free nerve endings surrounding the damaged fibers, resulting in localized pain and stiffness.

Despite the associated discomfort, DOMS is often regarded as a necessary part of exercise. For many, being sore creates the feeling that something is "happening" to their body—that they really accomplished something during their workout. And, on the surface, DOMS would seem to play at least some role in generating a training effect. Because DOMS is related to muscle damage and muscle damage is believed to initiate the growth process, it should follow that DOMS promotes muscular development. Makes sense, right?

The truth, however, is that DOMS is not a prerequisite for achieving results. Research shows that concentric-only exercise results in significant increases in lean muscle tissue without associated DOMS. Why is this relevant? Well, given the fact that DOMS is induced mainly from eccentric—not concentric—training, the natural conclusion is that soreness doesn't necessarily equate with progress.

So what is the lowdown on DOMS? When all is said and done, it's merely an indicator of tissue trauma—nothing more, nothing less. In the initial stages of training, the stimulus of exercise is a shock to your neuromuscular system. Your body doesn't know how to react to this stimulus, and the chain of events leading to muscular soreness is set into motion.

Unfortunately, there is little that can be done to prevent DOMS (outside of altering your training program). Warming up doesn't help. Neither does stretching. You can, however, alleviate soreness by engaging in an active recovery. Although the natural tendency is to remain sedentary if you are sore, this is counterproductive. Light activity is generally best, especially concentric-based activities. There also has been some research showing that postworkout massage can be of some help, but this seems to be dependent on the individual.

The good news is that the severity of DOMS will diminish over time. The human body is a very adaptive organism. It readily adjusts to the rigors of intense exercise—even after only a single bout of training. The muscles, connective tissue, and the immune system become increasingly efficient in dealing with fiber-related damage. Various physiologic and structural adaptations take place that gradually reduce any postexercise soreness. Thus, the more that you participate in regular exercise, the greater your resistance to muscle soreness.

The process can be compared to sunbathing. If you stay in the sun too long, your skin will burn. Shortly thereafter, the burn is accompanied by localized tissue swelling that is sensitive to pain. The burn heals over time and the skin becomes more resistant to the rays of the sun. Thereafter, repeated sun exposure results in a tan rather than a burn. While the specific adaptations in tanning are quite different than in training, the basic concept is the same: adaptation breeds resistance.

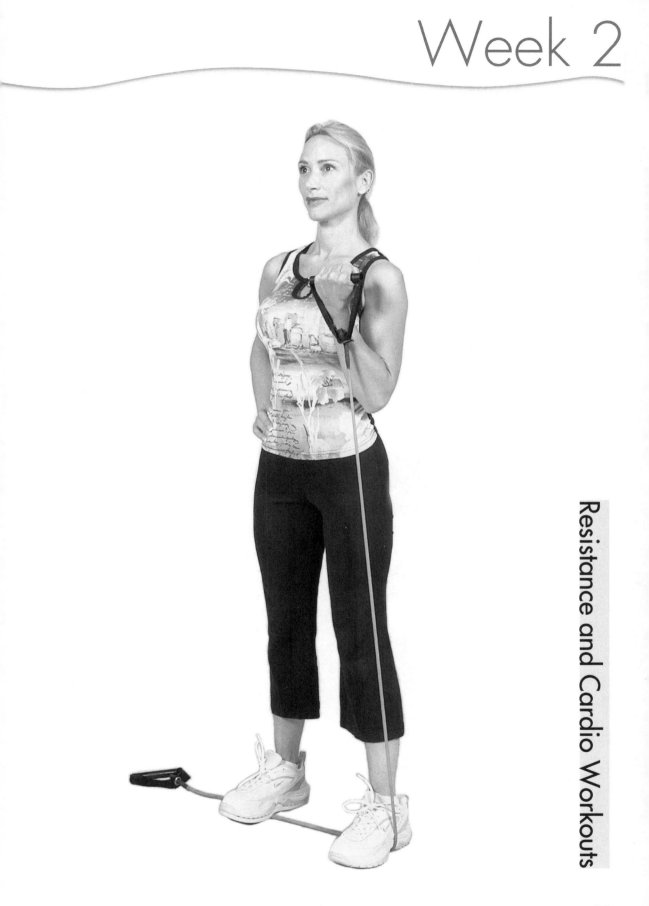

Resistance and Cardio Workouts

Day 8

Workout

Today will be a resistance workout. You'll train shoulders, biceps, and triceps. Exercises for shoulders will be performed in straight sets; exercises for biceps and triceps will be performed as supersets. Remember to selectively stretch the muscle group you are training between sets. Stretches for shoulders, triceps, and biceps are shown on pages 10, 11, and 12, respectively.

Gym	Sets	Reps	Home
Arnold Press 113	3	15 to 20	Arnold Press 113
One-Arm Cable Lateral Raise 116	3	15 to 20	One-Arm Strength Band Lateral Raise 117
Bench Rear Lateral Raise 119	3	15 to 20	Bench Rear Lateral Raise 119
Dumbbell Incline Curl 125	3	15 to 20	Dumbbell Incline Curl 125
Two-Arm Dumbbell Overhead Triceps Extension 143			Two-Arm Dumbbell Overhead Triceps Extension 143

Gym	Sets	Reps	Home
Dumbbell Hammer Curl 126	2	15 to 20	Dumbbell Hammer Curl 126
Triceps Dip 140			Triceps Dip 140
Prone Incline Curl 132	2	15 to 20	Prone Incline Curl 132
Nosebreaker 141			Two-Arm Dumbbell Lying Triceps Extension 141

Menu

Meal One

- 1 cup shredded wheat
- 4 ounces 1% milk

Meal Two

- Peach smoothie (containing 1 large peach, 1 scoop whey protein powder, 1 tablespoon flaxseed oil, and crushed ice)

Meal Three

- 6 ounces grilled chicken breast
- Large salad (containing romaine lettuce, green pepper, carrot, tomato, balsamic vinegar, and 1 tablespoon olive oil)

Meal Four

- 1 medium apple

Meal Five

- 6 ounces mahimahi
- 12 ounces zucchini

Day 9

Workout

Today will be a cardio workout. You'll be performing your training on the treadmill. I have provided target RPE intervals along with corresponding suggestions for enhancing intensity by varying the angle of incline and stride pace.

Minutes	RPE	Notes
3	3	Warm up at low intensity. No incline.
3	5	Slightly increase stride pace. No incline.
1	7	Increase stride pace. Increase the incline .5% every 30 seconds.
3	5	Decrease stride pace. Maintain current incline.
1	8	Increase stride pace. Increase the incline .5% every 30 seconds.
2	5	Decrease stride pace. Maintain current incline.
1	9	Increase stride pace. Increase the incline .5% every 30 seconds.
1	5	Decrease stride pace. Maintain current incline.
1	9	Increase stride pace. Increase the incline .5% every 30 seconds.
1	5	Decrease stride pace. Decrease the incline .5% every 30 seconds.
1	9	Increase stride pace. Maintain current incline.
2	5	Decrease stride pace. Decrease the incline .5% every 30 seconds.
1	8	Increase stride pace. Maintain current incline.
2	5	Decrease stride pace. Decrease the incline .5% every 30 seconds.
1	7	Increase stride pace. Maintain current incline.
3	5	Decrease stride pace. Decrease the incline .5% every 30 seconds.
3	3	Cool down at low intensity. No incline.

Day 9

Menu

Meal One

- 2 slices multigrain bread
- Mushroom omelet (containing 6 egg whites and 1 large portabella mushroom)
- 1 tablespoon flaxseed oil
- Coffee or tea

Meal Two

- Large plum

Meal Three

- Tuna salad (containing 6 ounces of tuna, mixed greens, and 1 tablespoon olive oil)
- 1 medium sweet potato

Meal Four

- 1 ounce raw, unsalted cashew nuts

Meal Five

- 4 ounces turkey breast
- 12 ounces cauliflower

Day 10

Workout

Today will be a resistance workout. You'll be training thighs (quadriceps), butt (glutes), and calves. Exercises for the quadriceps, butt, and hamstrings will be performed as supersets; exercises for the calves will be performed as straight sets. Remember to selectively stretch the muscle group you are training between sets. Stretches for glutes/hamstrings, quadriceps, and calves are on pages 12, 13, and 13, respectively.

Gym		Sets	Reps	Home	
Dumbbell Split-Squat Lunge	153	3	15 to 20	Dumbbell Split-Squat Lunge	153
Barbell Good Morning	163			Dumbbell Good Morning	162
Sissy Squat	154	3	15 to 20	Sissy Squat	154
Machine Lying Leg Curl	167			Weighted Lying Leg Curl	169
Machine Seated Adduction	155	3	15 to 20	Lying Adductor Raise	154
Machine Seated Abduction	173			Kneeling Abductor Raise	174

	Gym	Sets	Reps	Home	
One-Legged Toe Press	179	3	15 to 20	One-Legged Dumbbell Standing Calf Raise	181
Machine Seated Calf Raise	180	3	15 to 20	Dumbbell Seated Calf Raise	181

Menu

Meal One

- 1/2 cup oatmeal
- 1 scoop whey protein powder
- Coffee or tea

Meal Two

- Raspberry smoothie (containing 1 cup raspberries, 1 scoop whey protein powder, 1 tablespoon flaxseed oil, and crushed ice)

Meal Three

- 6 ounces grilled chicken breast
- Large salad (containing romaine lettuce, green pepper, carrot, tomato, balsamic vinegar, and 1 tablespoon olive oil)

Meal Four

- 1 cup diced pineapple

Meal Five

- 4 ounces grilled salmon
- 12 ounces collard greens

Day 11

Workout

Today will be a cardio workout. You'll be performing your training on the stationary bike. I have provided target RPE intervals along with corresponding suggestions for enhancing intensity by varying the resistance and/or pedal speed.

Minutes	RPE	Notes
3	3	Warm up at low resistance.
3	5	Slightly increase resistance and/or pedal speed.
1	7	Increase resistance and/or pedal speed.
3	5	Decrease resistance and/or pedal speed.
1	8	Increase resistance and/or pedal speed.
2	5	Decrease resistance and/or pedal speed.
1	9	Increase resistance and/or pedal speed.
1	5	Decrease resistance and/or pedal speed.
1	9	Increase resistance and/or pedal speed.
1	5	Decrease resistance and/or pedal speed.
1	9	Increase resistance and/or pedal speed.
2	5	Decrease resistance and/or pedal speed.
1	8	Increase resistance and/or pedal speed.
2	5	Decrease resistance and/or pedal speed.
1	7	Increase resistance and/or pedal speed.
3	5	Decrease resistance and/or pedal speed.
3	3	Cool down at low intensity.

Menu

Meal One

- 1 cup all-bran cereal
- 4 ounces 1% milk
- Coffee or tea

Meal Two

- 1 medium apple

Meal Three

- Turkey sandwich (containing 4 ounces sliced turkey breast on whole-wheat bread)
- Large salad (containing romaine lettuce, green pepper, carrot, tomato, onion, balsamic vinegar, and 1 tablespoon olive oil)

Meal Four

- 1 cup plain yogurt
- 1 tablespoon flaxseed oil

Meal Five

- 6 ounces filet of sole
- 12 ounces broccoli

Day 12

Workout

Today will be a resistance workout. You'll be training chest, back, and abdominals. Exercises for the chest and back will be performed as supersets; exercises for the abs will be performed as straight sets. Remember to selectively stretch the muscle group you are training between sets. Stretches for chest, back, and abdominals are on pages 10, 11, and 14, respectively.

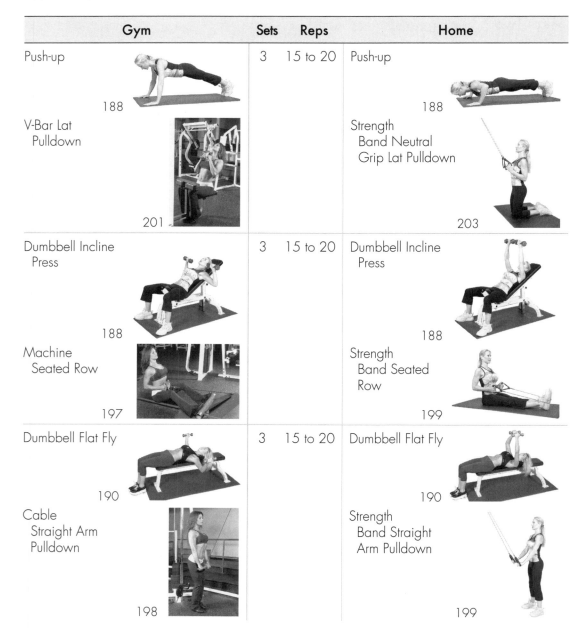

Gym	Sets	Reps	Home
Push-up 188	3	15 to 20	Push-up 188
V-Bar Lat Pulldown 201			Strength Band Neutral Grip Lat Pulldown 203
Dumbbell Incline Press 188	3	15 to 20	Dumbbell Incline Press 188
Machine Seated Row 197			Strength Band Seated Row 199
Dumbbell Flat Fly 190	3	15 to 20	Dumbbell Flat Fly 190
Cable Straight Arm Pulldown 198			Strength Band Straight Arm Pulldown 199

	Gym		Sets	Reps	Home	
Cable Kneeling Rope Crunch		213	3	15 to 20	Strength Band Kneeling Crunch	214
Leg Lowering		211	3	15 to 20	Leg Lowering	211

Menu

Meal One

- 6 ounces 1% cottage cheese
- 2 slices multigrain bread
- Coffee or tea

Meal Two

- 1 medium grapefruit

Meal Three

- 4 ounces grilled tofu
- Large salad (containing romaine lettuce, green pepper, carrot, tomato, onion, balsamic vinegar, and 1 tablespoon olive oil)

Meal Four

- Blueberry smoothie (containing 1 cup blueberries, 1 scoop whey protein powder, 1 tablespoon flaxseed oil, and crushed ice)

Meal Five

- 6 ounces sea bass
- 12 ounces green beans

Day 13

Workout

Today will be a cardio workout. You'll be performing your training on the stair climber. I have provided target RPE intervals along with corresponding suggestions for enhancing intensity by varying the resistance and/or step speed.

Minutes	RPE	Notes
3	3	Warm up at low intensity.
3	5	Slightly increase resistance and/or step speed.
1	7	Increase resistance and/or step speed.
3	5	Decrease resistance and/or step speed.
1	8	Increase resistance and/or step speed.
2	5	Decrease resistance and/or step speed.
1	9	Increase resistance and/or step speed.
1	5	Decrease resistance and/or step speed.
1	9	Increase resistance and/or step speed.
1	5	Decrease resistance and/or step speed.
1	9	Increase resistance and/or step speed.
2	5	Decrease resistance and/or step speed.
1	8	Increase resistance and/or step speed.
2	5	Decrease resistance and/or step speed.
1	7	Increase resistance and/or step speed.
3	5	Decrease resistance and/or step speed.
3	3	Cool down at low intensity.

Day 13

Menu

Meal One

- 2 slices multigrain bread
- Spanish omelet (containing 6 egg whites and 3 tablespoons salsa)
- 1 tablespoon flaxseed oil
- Coffee or tea

Meal Two

- 1 medium pear

Meal Three

- Tuna salad (containing 6 ounces of tuna, mixed greens, and 1 tablespoon olive oil)
- 1 medium sweet potato

Meal Four

- 1 ounce raw, unsalted walnuts

Meal Five

- 4 ounces broiled filet mignon
- 12 ounces asparagus

Day 14

Workout

Today is an off-day from training—a day to allow your body to recuperate from the intense training that you've done the rest of the week. Try to avoid any strenuous activities. If desired, you can do some light cardio such as walking. Most important—enjoy yourself!

Menu

Meal One

- 1/2 cup cream of wheat
- 1 scoop whey protein powder
- 1 tablespoon flaxseed oil
- Coffee or tea

Meal Two

- 1 ounce raw, unsalted peanuts

Meal Three

- 6 ounces grilled swordfish
- 1/2 cup brown rice

Meal Four

- 1/2 large papaya

Meal Five

- 4 ounces broiled extra-lean pork loin
- 12 ounces spinach

Week Three

4

You're now into your third week of the 28-Day Shapeover program and by this time you should be beginning to see some tangible changes in your physique. Your muscles should look and feel harder, your clothes should be fitting better, and your body should appear sleeker. In addition, you should feel more energized, with better endurance and more strength. You'll now build on these results and, by the end of the week, you should be close to attaining your monthly goal.

As in Week One, the resistance training protocol for this week will be focused on maximizing muscular development. You will be working to develop shapely muscles that enhance your symmetry and stoke your metabolism. New techniques will be introduced to further these objectives.

Let's go over the protocol in detail.

Resistance Training Protocol

Sets　During Week Three, you will perform two to four sets of each exercise. The sets will be executed in a straight fashion, meaning you do a set, rest for the prescribed amount of time, do another set, rest, and so on. Make sure to perform the desired number of sets for a particular movement before moving on the next exercise.

To jack up workout intensity, you will perform a *double drop set* on the final set of each exercise. Simply stated, this means that after you have performed the target number of reps, you drop the weight by approximately 25 to 30 percent and then perform as many additional reps as you can; then, when you are not able to complete any more reps at the reduced weight, you drop the weight again by approximately 25 to 30 percent and rep out for whatever you can get. For example, say you perform a dumbbell chest press with 20 pounds. In the drop set, you'll begin with 20-pound dumbbells for the prescribed number of repetitions, immediately drop down to the 15-pound dumbbells for as many reps as you can get, and then drop down to the 10-pound dumbbells to muscular failure. In this way, you are able to exhaust a muscle beyond what is otherwise possible, shocking its fibers into further development. After completing a drop set, you'll soon see why they're often called "burn sets"!

Remember, though, you should only perform the drops on your final set of each exercise. The ultra-intense nature of this technique really depletes your body's resources. Overdo it with too many drop sets and you can easily become overtrained, thereby setting back your progress (see the sidebar on overtraining for more details about this phenomenon).

Repetitions   During Week Three, you will use a moderate repetition scheme, aiming for 8 to 10 reps per set. You will again be looking to stimulate the full range of muscle fibers, especially the strength-oriented type II fibers, as well as maximizing cellular hydration and hormonal release.

As previously noted, the only exception to the moderate rep protocol is for the performance of seated calf raises. Because this exercise targets the soleus muscle, which is comprised almost predominantly of slow-twitch muscle fibers, it responds better to a higher rep scheme. Therefore, you'll perform 15 to 20 reps on this movement.

Rest Intervals   During Week Three, you will take approximately 60 to 90 seconds between sets. Because the goal is strength and hypertrophy and the weights are moderately heavy, this will allow enough time for adequate recovery from the previous set.

As always, you will employ selective muscular stretching between each set, stretching the muscle that is being worked. Again, stretch statically, easing into each move in a slow, controlled fashion.

Cardio Protocol

The cardio component for this week will again kick exercise intensity up a notch. The low-intensity intervals will be further reduced and your rating of perceived exertion will increase.

You'll start with a warm-up and then, after a lone 3:1 low-intensity interval, the next intervals will go from a ratio of 2:1 down to 1:1. On your higher-intensity intervals, you will also spend a greater amount of time at an RPE of 9. The intervals conclude with a mild cool-down. If the protocol becomes too intense, simply do what you can; remember, aerobic capacity improves over time and, provided you keep up with the routine, you'll ultimately reach the goal.

I have suggested the treadmill, stair climber, and stationary bike as the modalities of choice, but feel free to substitute alternative exercises at your discretion. If possible, try to cross-train using at least two different movements from session to session to allow for sufficient variety.

Understanding Overtraining

Overtraining syndrome (OTS) is a common exercise-related affliction. Studies show that it affects as much as 10 percent of all people who exercise on a regular basis. Because of a lack of understanding about the subject, it often ends up going undiagnosed.

Simply stated, overtraining results from performing too much strenuous physical activity. However, the exact threshold for overtraining varies from person to person. Everyone responds differently to exercise. Some people can tolerate large volumes of training while others much less. What's more, factors such as nutritional status, sleeping patterns, hormonal and enzymatic concentrations, muscle fiber composition, and previous training experience all affect recuperative capacity and, therefore, the point at which overtraining rears its ugly head.

Overtraining can be classified into two separate categories: localized and systemic. Although both have the same origin (too much exercise), their repercussions are quite different. Of the two subtypes, localized overtraining is by far the most common. As the name implies, it is localized to a specific muscle or muscle group without affecting other bodily systems. It generally strikes those who are involved in serious strength training programs, especially bodybuilders, powerlifters, and fitness competitors.

Localized overtraining is bound to occur when the same muscle group is trained too frequently in a given time span. This can even happen in a split routine, where different muscle groups are trained on different days (my shapeover program employs a split routine). You see, during the performance of most exercises, there is a synergistic interaction between muscle groups. The biceps, for instance, are integrally involved in the performance of back maneuvers; the shoulders and triceps are involved in many exercises for the chest, as are the glutes and hamstrings during compound leg movements. Other muscles function as stabilizers: the abdominals and erector spinae (the muscles of the lower back), in particular, help to provide stability in a variety of upper- and lower-body exercises, contracting statically throughout each move. The fact is, when a muscle is repeatedly subjected to intense physical stress (even on a secondary level) without being afforded adequate rest, the rate at which microtrauma occurs outpaces the reparation process. The end result: impaired localized muscular development.

Systemic overtraining, on the other hand, is more complex, and potentially more serious, than localized overtraining. As the name implies, it is all-encompassing, acting on the body as a whole. Commonly referred to as overtraining syndrome (OTS, for short), it affects thousands of people each year. Both strength and endurance athletes are equally at risk.

In almost all cases, OTS causes the body to enter a catabolic state. Catabolism is mediated by an increased production of cortisol—a stress hormone secreted by the adrenal cortex—which exerts its influence at the cellular level, impeding muscular repair and function. Making matters worse, there often is a corresponding decrease in testosterone production, depleting the body of its most potent anabolic stimulus. Together, these factors combine to inhibit protein synthesis and accelerate proteolysis (protein breakdown). Not only does this result in a cessation of muscular development, but it also makes the body less efficient at utilizing fat for fuel—a double whammy that wreaks havoc on body composition.

In addition, because of a depletion of glutamine stores, OTS suppresses the body's immune system. Glutamine is the major source of energy for immune cells. A steady supply is necessary for their proper function. However, glutamine levels are rapidly exhausted when exercise volume is high. Without an adequate amount of fuel, the immune system loses its ability to produce antibodies such as lymphocytes, leukocytes, and cytokines. Ultimately, the body's capacity to fight viral and bacterial infections becomes impaired, leading to an increased incidence of infirmity.

Below are some of the symptoms related to overtraining. If you experience two or more of these symptoms, you very well might be overtrained. If symptoms persist, get plenty of sleep and don't resume training until you feel mentally and physically ready.

- Increased resting heart rate
- Increased resting blood pressure
- Decreased exercise performance
- Decreased appetite
- Decreased desire to work out
- Increased incidence of injuries
- Increased incidence of infections and flulike symptoms
- Increased irritability and depression

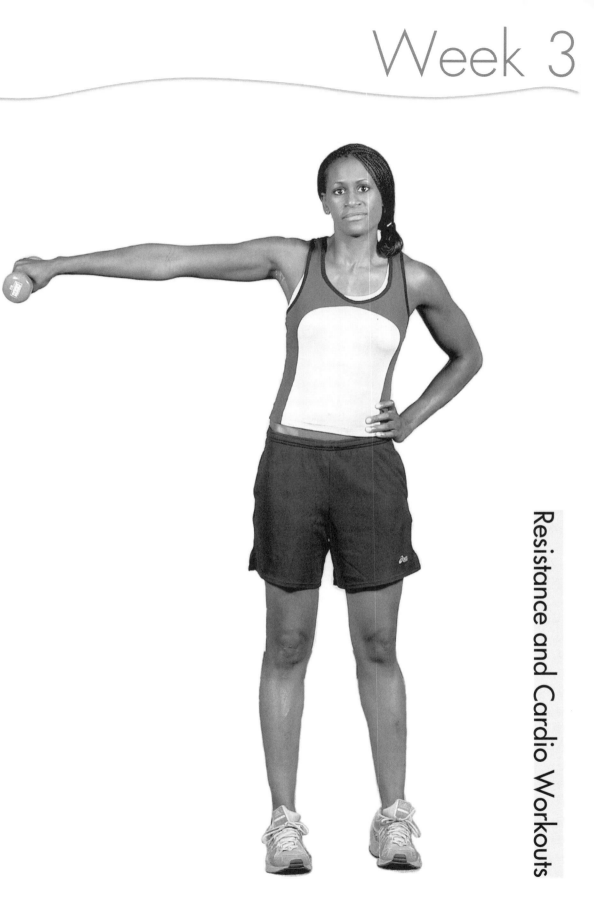

Day 15

Workout

Today will be a resistance workout. You'll train shoulders, biceps, and triceps. On the last set of each exercise, you will perform a double drop set, proceeding to muscular fatigue. Remember to selectively stretch the muscle group you are training between sets. Stretches for shoulders, triceps, and biceps are shown on pages 10, 11, and 12, respectively.

Gym		Sets	Reps	Home	
Machine Shoulder Press	120	4	8 to 10	Dumbbell Shoulder Press	113
One-Arm Dumbbell Lateral Raise	122	3	8 to 10	One-Arm Dumbbell Lateral Raise	122
Machine Rear Lateral	121	3	8 to 10	Dumbbell Bent Lateral Raise	119
Seated Dumbbell Curl	124	3	8 to 10	Seated Dumbbell Curl	124
One-Arm Cable Rope Hammer Curl	128	2	8 to 10	One-Arm Strength Band Hammer Curl	134
Barbell Preacher Curl	133	2	8 to 10	One-Arm Dumbbell Bench Preacher Curl	131

Gym	Sets	Reps	Home
One-Arm Dumbbell Lying Triceps Extension 145	3	8 to 10	One-Arm Dumbbell Lying Triceps Extension 145
Machine Triceps Extension 142	3	8 to 10	Strength Band Overhead Triceps Extension 145
Cable Triceps Kickback 138	2	8 to 10	Strength Band Triceps Kickback 147

Menu

Meal One

- 6 ounces 1% cottage cheese
- 2 slices multigrain bread
- Coffee or tea

Meal Two

- 1 cup diced mango

Meal Three

- 4 ounces grilled turkey breast
- Large salad (containing romaine lettuce, green pepper, carrot, tomato, onion, balsamic vinegar, and 1 tablespoon olive oil)

Meal Four

- Blueberry smoothie (containing 1 cup blueberries, 1 scoop whey protein powder, 1 tablespoon flaxseed oil, and crushed ice)

Meal Five

- 6 ounces broiled red snapper
- 12 ounces string beans

Day 16

Workout

Today will be a cardio workout. You'll be performing your training on the treadmill. I have provided target RPE intervals along with corresponding suggestions for enhancing intensity by varying the angle of incline and stride pace.

Minutes	RPE	Notes
3	3	Warm up at low intensity. No incline.
3	5	Slightly increase stride pace. No incline.
1	7	Increase stride pace. Increase the incline .5% every 30 seconds.
2	5	Decrease stride pace. Maintain current incline.
1	8	Increase stride pace. Increase the incline .5% every 30 seconds.
2	5	Decrease stride pace. Maintain current incline.
1	9	Increase stride pace. Increase the incline .5% every 30 seconds.
1	5	Decrease stride pace. Maintain current incline.
1	9	Increase stride pace. Increase the incline .5% every 30 seconds.
1	5	Decrease stride pace. Maintain current incline.
1	9	Increase stride pace. Increase the incline .5% every 30 seconds.
1	5	Decrease stride pace. Decrease the incline .5% every 30 seconds.
1	9	Increase stride pace. Maintain current incline.
2	5	Decrease stride pace. Decrease the incline .5% every 30 seconds.
1	9	Increase stride pace. Maintain current incline.
2	5	Decrease stride pace. Decrease the incline .5% every 30 seconds.
1	8	Increase stride pace. Maintain current incline.
2	5	Decrease stride pace. Decrease the incline .5% every 30 seconds.
3	3	Cool down at low intensity. No incline.

Menu

Meal One

- 1 cup cream of wheat
- 1 scoop whey protein powder
- 1 tablespoon flaxseed oil
- Coffee or tea

Meal Two

- 1 cup strawberries

Meal Three

- 4 ounces chicken breast
- 1/2 cup brown rice

Meal Four

- 1 cup plain yogurt

Meal Five

- 4 ounces broiled sirloin steak
- 12 ounces asparagus
- 1 tablespoon olive oil

Day 17

Workout

Today will be a resistance workout. You'll be training thighs (quadriceps), butt (glutes), and calves. On the last set of each exercise, you will perform a double drop set, proceeding to muscular fatigue. Remember to selectively stretch the muscle group you are training between sets. Stretches for glutes/hamstrings, quadriceps, and calves are on pages 12, 13, and 13, respectively.

Gym		Sets	Reps	Home	
Step Up	159	4	8 to 10	Step Up	159
One-Legged Machine Leg Extension	151	3	8 to 10	One-Legged Weighted Leg Extension	153
Cable Standing Adductor Raise	160	3	8 to 10	Lying Leg Cross	159
Butt Blaster	164	3	8 to 10	Floor Kick	165
Machine Kneeling Leg Curl	168	3	8 to 10	One-Legged Weighted Lying Leg Curl	169
Prone Hip Extension	165	2	8 to 10	Prone Hip Extension	165

	Gym	Sets	Reps	Home	
One-Legged Machine Standing Calf Raise	182	3	8 to 10	One-Legged Dumbbell Standing Calf Raise	181
One-Legged Machine Seated Calf Raise	177	3	15 to 20	One-Legged Dumbbell Seated Calf Raise	178

Menu

Meal One

- 1 cup muesli cereal
- 4 ounces 1% milk

Meal Two

- Peach smoothie (containing 1 medium peach, 1 scoop whey protein powder, 1 tablespoon flaxseed oil, and crushed ice)

Meal Three

- 6 ounces grilled ahi tuna steak
- Large salad (containing romaine lettuce, green pepper, carrot, tomato, balsamic vinegar, and 1 tablespoon olive oil)

Meal Four

- 1 ounce raw, unsalted macadamia nuts

Meal Five

- 1 pound steamed lobster
- 12 ounces Chinese vegetable stir-fry

Day 18

Workout

Today will be a cardio workout. You'll be performing your training on the stationary bike. I have provided target RPE intervals along with corresponding suggestions for enhancing intensity by varying the resistance and/or pedal speed.

Minutes	RPE	Notes
3	3	Warm up at low intensity.
3	5	Slightly increase resistance and/or pedal speed.
1	7	Increase resistance and/or pedal speed.
2	5	Decrease resistance and/or pedal speed.
1	8	Increase resistance and/or pedal speed.
2	5	Decrease resistance and/or pedal speed.
1	9	Increase resistance and/or pedal speed.
1	5	Decrease resistance and/or pedal speed.
1	9	Increase resistance and/or pedal speed.
1	5	Decrease resistance and/or pedal speed.
1	9	Increase resistance and/or pedal speed.
1	5	Decrease resistance and/or pedal speed.
1	9	Increase resistance and/or pedal speed.
2	5	Decrease resistance and/or pedal speed.
1	9	Increase resistance and/or pedal speed.
2	5	Decrease resistance and/or pedal speed.
1	8	Increase resistance and/or pedal speed.
2	5	Decrease resistance and/or pedal speed.
3	3	Cool down at low intensity.

Day 18

Menu

Meal One

- 2 slices multigrain bread
- Spinach omelet (containing 6 egg whites and chopped spinach)
- 1 tablespoon flaxseed oil
- Coffee or tea

Meal Two

- 2 slices pineapple

Meal Three

- 4 ounces grilled extra-lean pork loin
- 1/4 cup long-grain brown rice (measured uncooked)

Meal Four

- 1 ounce walnuts

Meal Five

- 4 ounces broiled halibut steak
- 12 ounces summer squash

Day 19

Workout

Today will be a resistance workout. You'll be training chest, back, and abdominals. On the last set of each exercise, you will perform a double drop set, proceeding to muscular fatigue. Remember to selectively stretch the muscle group you are training between sets. Stretches for chest, back, and abdominals are on pages 10, 11, and 14, respectively.

Gym		Sets	Reps	Home	
Machine Flat Press	192	4	8 to 10	Dumbbell Flat Press	187
Barbell Incline Press	186	3	8 to 10	Dumbbell Incline Press	188
Cable High Pulley Crossover	193	3	8 to 10	Dumbbell Incline Fly	190
Assisted Chin-Up	205	4	8 to 10	Strength Band Reverse Lat Pulldown	206
One-Arm Cable Standing Low Row	208	3	8 to 10	One-Arm Strength Band Standing Low Row	209
Cross Cable Pulldown	207	3	8 to 10	Strength Band High Lat Pull	209

Day 19

	Gym		Sets	Reps	Home	
Toe Touch		216	3	8 to 10	Toe Touch	216
Pedaling		216	3	8 to 10	Pedaling	216

Menu

Meal One

- 1/2 cup oatmeal
- 1 scoop whey protein powder
- Coffee or tea

Meal Two

- Blackberry smoothie (containing 1 cup blackberries, 1 scoop whey protein powder, 1 tablespoon flaxseed oil, and crushed ice)

Meal Three

- 6 ounces broiled filet of flounder
- Large salad (containing romaine lettuce, green pepper, carrot, tomato, balsamic vinegar, and 1 tablespoon olive oil)

Meal Four

- 1 ounce raw, unsalted mixed nuts

Meal Five

- 4 ounces grilled salmon
- 12 ounces collard greens

Day 20

Workout

Today will be a cardio workout. You'll be performing your training on the stair climber. I have provided target RPE intervals along with corresponding suggestions for enhancing intensity by varying the resistance and/or step speed.

Minutes	RPE	Notes
3	3	Warm up at low intensity.
3	5	Slightly increase resistance and/or step speed.
1	7	Increase resistance and/or step speed.
2	5	Decrease resistance and/or step speed.
1	8	Increase resistance and/or step speed.
2	5	Decrease resistance and/or step speed.
1	9	Increase resistance and/or step speed.
1	5	Decrease resistance and/or step speed.
1	9	Increase resistance and/or step speed.
1	5	Decrease resistance and/or step speed.
1	9	Increase resistance and/or step speed.
1	5	Decrease resistance and/or step speed.
1	9	Increase resistance and/or step speed.
2	5	Decrease resistance and/or step speed.
1	9	Increase resistance and/or step speed.
2	5	Decrease resistance and/or step speed.
1	8	Increase resistance and/or step speed.
2	5	Decrease resistance and/or step speed.
3	3	Cool down at low intensity.

Menu

Meal One

- 1 cup all-bran cereal
- 4 ounces 1% milk
- Coffee or tea

Meal Two

- 1 ounce raw, unsalted pecan nuts

Meal Three

- Roast beef sandwich (containing 4 ounces lean, sliced roast beef on multigrain bread)
- Large salad (containing romaine lettuce, green pepper, carrot, tomato, onion, balsamic vinegar, and 1 tablespoon olive oil)

Meal Four

- 1 cup plain yogurt
- 1 tablespoon flaxseed oil

Meal Five

- 4 ounces broiled shark steak
- 12 ounces kale

Day 21

Workout

Today is an off-day from training—a day to allow your body to recuperate from the intense training that you've done the rest of the week. Try to avoid any strenuous activities. If desired, you can do some light cardio such as walking. Most important—enjoy yourself!

Menu

Meal One

- Tex-Mex omelet (containing 6 egg whites and chopped onion, tomato, green pepper, and jalapeno pepper)
- 1 tablespoon flaxseed oil
- Coffee or tea

Meal Two

- 1 ounce raw, unsalted almonds

Meal Three

- Black bean salad (containing 4 ounces black beans, lettuce, tomato, and cucumber with light vinaigrette dressing).

Meal Four

- 1 cup cubed cantaloupe

Meal Five

- 4 ounces broiled venison
- 12 ounces okra

5

Week Four

You are entering Week Four—the final week—of the 28-Day Shapeover program. You should now see some fairly significant changes in your body at this point. Your clothes should be fitting better, your muscles should be harder, and you should feel stronger and more energetic.

In this final week, you'll be honing your muscles still further with endurance-based toning workouts. The intensity of the routine will be ratcheted up significantly with the inclusion of a specialized technique called giant sets. You'll really push yourself here but it will all pay off in the end.

Let's go over the protocol for Week Four in detail.

Resistance Training Protocol

Sets   You will perform three sets of each exercise. For all muscle groups except the calves, the sets will be executed as giant sets. A *giant set* is any set that incorporates three or more different exercises in succession. You move directly from one exercise to the next, without resting in between movements. This not only heightens exercise intensity (and thus muscle development), but also creates an aerobic environment, thereby expediting fat burning.

You will perform giant sets for the same muscle group. For example, in Day 22, you will begin by performing a front raise; then, upon completing the specified number of reps, go immediately to the lateral raise for the specified number of reps, and then immediately to the bent lateral. After a brief rest, you will repeat the process, rest again, and repeat the process a final time. Then you will move on to giant sets for your biceps and triceps.

As previously mentioned, the only muscle group that is excluded from giant sets is the calves. Because of their physiologic composition, only two moves are necessary to fully activate this muscle complex, making giant sets superfluous. Thus, you will perform a superset for the calves, alternating between standing and seated calf raises (i.e., perform a set of standing calf raises and then move immediately to the seated calf raise, rest, repeat, rest, repeat).

Repetitions   Since this week's focus is on honing muscle tone and endurance, you will utilize a high rep scheme, aiming for 15 to 20 reps per set. This targets the slow-twitch muscle fibers that, despite their lack of growth potential, make a significant contribution to the quality of your muscle tone and help to produce a sleek, hard physique.

Of course, you must choose a weight that challenges your muscles. If you are getting to 20 reps and can easily do a few more, then the weight is too light. Remember, intensity is the most important determinant in body sculpting; make sure you don't take the easy way out!

Rest Intervals   You will keep your rest intervals to a minimum, taking no more than 30 seconds between giant sets (there should be little or no rest between exercises during a giant set).

As a rule, training should commence before you can fully catch your breath. This will create a distinct aerobic effect, keeping your heart rate elevated throughout the session. This results in a substantial increase in caloric expenditure, ultimately helping to elevate metabolism and reduce body fat. As always, you will employ selective muscular stretching between each giant set, stretching the muscle that is being worked.

Cardio Protocol

The cardio component for this week will, once again, up exercise intensity from the preceding week. The low-intensity intervals will be still further reduced and your rating of perceived exertion will increase even more. Plan to really work up a sweat!

You'll start with a warm-up and then proceed to a lone 3:1 low-intensity interval before alternating the rest of the way on a 1:1 basis. The high-intensity intervals will predominantly be done at an RPE of 9. The intervals will conclude with a mild cool-down. If the protocol becomes too intense, simply do what you can and strive to do a little more in your next cardio session.

I have suggested the treadmill, stair climber, and stationary bike as the modalities of choice, but feel free to substitute alternative exercises at your discretion. If possible, try to cross-train using at least two different movements from session to session to allow for sufficient variety.

Understanding Compound and Isolation Movements

It's important to note that my shapeover program uses a fairly balanced mix of both compound and isolation movements. For those who aren't familiar with these terms, here's a brief overview.

As a rule, a compound movement involves the action of two joints, whereas an isolation movement only involves one joint. Consequently, many supporting muscles are involved in the completion of a compound movement. Certain compound movements, like the Olympic deadlift, require virtually all of the major muscles of the body to be utilized in exercise performance. On the other hand, isolation movements tend to target a specific muscle or muscle group at the exclusion of secondary muscles. Because only one joint is used to lift a weight, rarely will supporting muscles come into play in exercise performance.

For example, the squat is a compound movement because both the knee and hip joints are utilized in order to complete a repetition. As you descend into a squat position, both your knees and hips bend in order to allow your body to move downward. Conversely, a leg extension is an isolation movement because only the knee joint is utilized in performance. Although both exercises primarily stress the quadriceps, they exert stimulus to different areas of the lower body. In most variations of the squat, you stimulate all the muscles of the quadriceps and provide secondary stress to the muscles of the glutes and hamstrings and even the calves. In effect, your entire lower body is worked in this exercise. On the other hand, the leg extension almost exclusively stresses the muscles in the lower part of the quadriceps, particularly in the area of the knee (vastus medialis and vastus lateralis). You provide secondary stress to the upper portion of the quadriceps (rectus femoris) and virtually no stress to the hamstrings and glutes. Hence, understanding the complexities of compound and isolation exercises is paramount to your training goals. Here's why it's essential to include both types of movements for body sculpting purposes:

Compound movements are the "meat and potatoes" of your routine. They help to develop your proportions in a way that would be impossible solely by using isolation exercises. The benefits of these movements include:

- *They strengthen the connective tissue that supports your muscles.* If your connective tissue is sufficiently weaker than your muscle tissue, you are more prone to tendon and ligament injuries such as strains, tears, and tendonitis. What's more, your connective tissue works in conjunction with your muscles and must be strong to train at high levels of intensity.

- *They help to stimulate many of the smaller, stabilizer muscles that are not specifically targeted by most exercises.* Many of the smaller muscles of the body are not involved in the execution of single joint movements. These smaller muscles assist in exercise performance and thus help to shape the larger muscles. Moreover, they help to add overall detail to your physique and give your body a polished appearance.

- *They maximize EPOC.* Because compound movements involve many different muscle groups, they require much greater oxygen utilization. This ultimately increases the amount of calories you burn post-workout, promoting a leaner physique.

Isolation movements allow you to target specific muscles. An isolation movement requires the use of lighter weights than a compound movement. Because supporting muscles are not involved in the movement, the target muscle has to perform almost all of the work. As a rule, you should be able to perform about 50 percent of the weight used in a compound movement for the same muscle group. This can vary somewhat based on the strength of your primary muscle in a particular exercise. The benefits of isolation movements include:

- *They can selectively target a muscle at the exclusion of secondary muscles.* The degree to which you can isolate a particular muscle is somewhat limited. It is influenced by where the muscle is situated on your body and the range of motion of the movement itself. Nevertheless, single-joint exercises are much more concentrated to an individual muscle. Thus, isolation movements tend to be better for body sculpting and creating muscular symmetry.

- *They put less stress on the connective tissue in comparison to compound movements.* Because the amount of weight that you can utilize is substantially less than for compound movements, isolation exercises reduce the tension applied to the tendons and joints. Hence, they help to decrease the chance of injury to the connective tissue, which is one of the most common training-related ailments. This can be of particular benefit when you are training around a previous injury or medical debility.

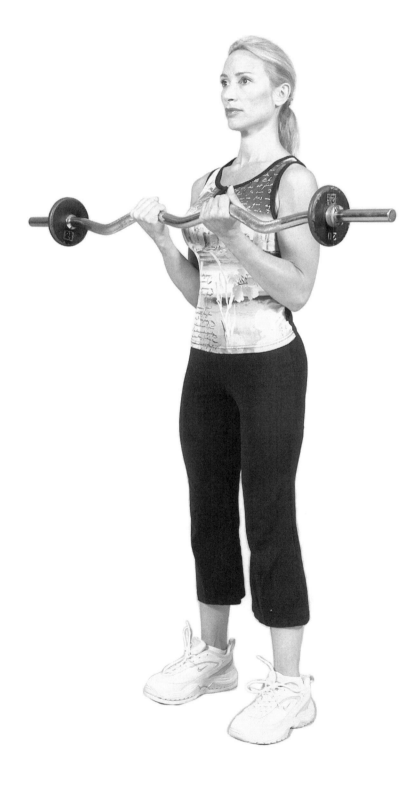

Day 22

Workout

Today will be a resistance workout. You'll train shoulders, biceps, and triceps. All exercises will be performed as giant sets. Remember to selectively stretch the muscle group you are training between each giant set. Stretches for shoulders, triceps, and biceps are shown on pages 10, 11, and 12, respectively.

Gym		Sets	Reps	Home	
Dumbbell Front Raise	114	3	15 to 20	Dumbbell Front Raise	114
Dumbbell Lateral Raise	117			Dumbbell Lateral Raise	117
Dumbbell Bent Lateral Raise	119			Dumbbell Bent Lateral Raise	119
EZ Curl	126	3	15 to 20	Dumbbell Incline Curl	125
Cable Rope Hammer Curl	127			Dumbbell Hammer Curl	126
Machine Preacher Curl	130			One-Arm Dumbbell Bench Preacher Curl	131

Gym	Sets	Reps	Home
Cable Rope Pressdown 136	3	15 to 20	Strength Band Pressdown 137
Standing Cable Overhead Rope Triceps Extension 144			Two-Arm Dumbbell Overhead Triceps Extension 143
Machine Overhead Triceps Extension 146			Two-Arm Dumbbell Lying Triceps Extension 141

Menu

Meal One

- 1 cup bran flakes cereal
- 4 ounces 1% milk
- Coffee or tea

Meal Two

- Grape smoothie (containing 1 cup seedless grapes, 1 scoop whey protein powder, 1 tablespoon flaxseed oil, and crushed ice)

Meal Three

- 6 ounces grilled chicken breast
- Large salad (containing romaine lettuce, green pepper, carrot, tomato, balsamic vinegar, and 1 tablespoon olive oil)

Meal Four

- 1 ounce raw, unsalted almonds

Meal Five

- 6 ounces broiled grouper
- 12 ounces cauliflower

Day 23

Workout

Today will be a cardio workout. You'll be performing your training on the treadmill. I have provided target RPE intervals along with corresponding suggestions for enhancing intensity by varying the angle of incline and stride pace.

Minutes	RPE	Notes
3	3	Warm up at low intensity. No incline.
2	5	Slightly increase stride pace. No incline.
1	7	Increase stride pace. Increase the incline .5% every 30 seconds.
1	5	Decrease stride pace. Maintain current incline.
1	8	Increase stride pace. Increase the incline .5% every 30 seconds.
1	5	Decrease stride pace. Maintain current incline.
1	9	Increase stride pace. Increase the incline .5% every 30 seconds.
1	5	Decrease stride pace. Maintain current incline.
1	9	Increase stride pace. Increase the incline .5% every 30 seconds.
1	5	Decrease stride pace. Maintain current incline.
1	9	Increase stride pace. Increase the incline .5% every 30 seconds.
1	5	Decrease stride pace. Maintain current incline.
1	9	Increase stride pace. Increase the incline .5% every 30 seconds.
1	5	Decrease stride pace. Decrease the incline .5% every 30 seconds.
1	9	Increase stride pace. Maintain current incline.
1	5	Decrease stride pace. Decrease the incline .5% every 30 seconds.
1	9	Increase stride pace. Maintain current incline.
1	5	Decrease stride pace. Decrease the incline .5% every 30 seconds.
1	9	Increase stride pace. Maintain current incline.
1	5	Decrease stride pace. Decrease the incline .5% every 30 seconds.
1	8	Increase stride pace. Maintain current incline.
1	5	Decrease stride pace. Decrease the incline .5% every 30 seconds.
1	7	Increase stride pace. Maintain current incline.
1	5	Decrease stride pace. Decrease the incline .5% every 30 seconds.
3	3	Cool down at low intensity. No incline.

Menu

Meal One

- 1/2 cup oatmeal
- 1 scoop whey protein powder
- 1 tablespoon flaxseed oil
- Coffee or tea

Meal Two

- 1 ounce raw, unsalted walnuts

Meal Three

- Chicken sandwich (containing 4 ounces sliced chicken breast on rye bread)
- Large salad (containing romaine lettuce, green pepper, carrot, tomato, onion, balsamic vinegar, and 1 tablespoon olive oil)

Meal Four

- 1 cup cubed honeydew melon

Meal Five

- 6 ounces broiled shrimp
- 12 ounces spinach

Day 24

Workout

Today will be a resistance workout. You'll be training thighs (quadriceps), butt (glutes), and calves. Exercises for the quadriceps and butt will be performed as giant sets; exercises for the calves will be performed as supersets. Remember to selectively stretch the muscle group you are training between sets. Stretches for glutes/hamstrings, quadriceps, and calves are on pages 12, 13, and 13, respectively.

Gym		Sets	Reps	Home	
Machine Leg Press	157	3	15 to 20	Dumbbell Squat	152
Jump Squat	158			Jump Squat	158
Machine Leg Extension	156			Weighted Leg Extension	158
Barbell Good Morning	163	3	15 to 20	Dumbbell Good Morning	162
Machine Seated Leg Curl	170			Weighted Lying Leg Curl	169
Lying Abductor Raise	172			Lying Abductor Raise	172

	Gym		Sets	Reps	Home	
Toe Press	183		3	15 to 20	Dumbbell Standing Calf Raise	178
Machine Seated Calf Raise	180				Dumbbell Seated Calf Raise	181

Menu

Meal One

- 6 ounces 1% cottage cheese
- 2 slices multigrain bread
- Coffee or tea

Meal Two

- 1 ounce raw, unsalted pistachio nuts

Meal Three

- 4 ounces grilled turkey breast
- Large salad (containing romaine lettuce, green pepper, carrot, tomato, onion, balsamic vinegar, and 1 tablespoon olive oil)

Meal Four

- Kiwi smoothie (containing 2 kiwis, 1 scoop whey protein powder, 1 tablespoon flaxseed oil, and crushed ice)

Meal Five

- 6 ounces broiled codfish
- 12 ounces Chinese stir-fried vegetables

Day 25

Workout

Today will be a cardio workout. You'll be performing your training on the stationary bike. I have provided target RPE intervals along with corresponding suggestions for enhancing intensity by varying the resistance and/or pedal speed.

Minutes	RPE	Notes
3	3	Warm up at low intensity.
2	5	Slightly increase resistance and/or pedal speed.
1	7	Increase resistance and/or pedal speed.
1	5	Decrease resistance and/or pedal speed.
1	8	Increase resistance and/or pedal speed.
1	5	Decrease resistance and/or pedal speed.
1	9	Increase resistance and/or pedal speed.
1	5	Decrease resistance and/or pedal speed.
1	9	Increase resistance and/or pedal speed.
1	5	Decrease resistance and/or pedal speed.
1	9	Increase resistance and/or pedal speed.
1	5	Decrease resistance and/or pedal speed.
1	9	Increase resistance and/or pedal speed.
1	5	Decrease resistance and/or pedal speed.
1	9	Increase resistance and/or pedal speed.
1	5	Decrease resistance and/or pedal speed.
1	9	Increase resistance and/or pedal speed.
1	5	Decrease resistance and/or pedal speed.
1	9	Increase resistance and/or pedal speed.
1	5	Decrease resistance and/or pedal speed.
1	8	Increase resistance and/or pedal speed.
1	5	Decrease resistance and/or pedal speed.
1	7	Increase resistance and/or pedal speed.
1	5	Decrease resistance and/or pedal speed.
3	3	Cool down at low intensity.

Menu

Meal One

- 1 cup cream of wheat
- 1 tablespoon flaxseed oil
- 1 scoop whey protein powder
- Coffee or tea

Meal Two

- 1 medium apple

Meal Three

- 4 ounces broiled sea bass
- 1 medium sweet potato

Meal Four

- 1 cup plain yogurt

Meal Five

- 4 ounces grilled London broil
- 12 ounces green beans

Day 26

Workout

Today will be a resistance workout. You'll be training chest, back, and abdominals. All exercises will be performed as giant sets. Remember to selectively stretch the muscle group you are training between sets. Stretches for chest, back, and abdominals are on pages 10, 11, and 14, respectively.

Gym		Sets	Reps	Home	
Machine Incline Chest Press	189	3	15 to 20	Dumbbell Incline Press	188
Dumbbell Flat Fly	190			Dumbbell Flat Fly	190
Cable Low Pulley Crossover	191			Push-up	188
Front Lat Pulldown	195	3	15 to 20	Strength Band Overhand Lat Pulldown	206
Cable Standing Reverse Low Row	202			One-Arm Dumbbell Row	196
Dumbbell Pullover	196			Dumbbell Pullover	196

	Gym	Sets	Reps	Home	
Crunch		3	15 to 20	Crunch	
	214				214
Reverse Curl				Reverse Curl	
	215				215
Side Jackknife				Side Jackknife	
	215				215

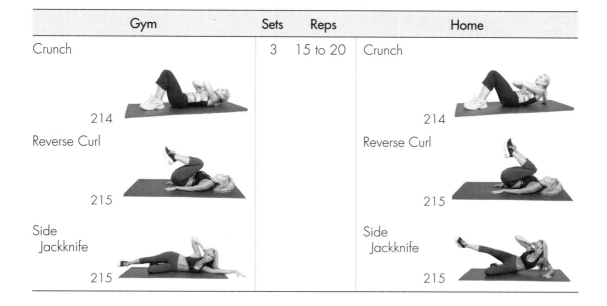

Menu

Meal One

- 1 cup Kashi cereal
- 4 ounces 1% milk

Meal Two

- Banana smoothie (containing 1 medium banana, 1 scoop whey protein powder, 1 tablespoon flax-seed oil, and crushed ice)

Meal Three

- Turkey burger (containing 6 ounces ground turkey breast on whole-wheat roll)
- Large salad (containing romaine lettuce, green pepper, carrot, tomato, balsamic vinegar, and 1 tablespoon olive oil)

Meal Four

- 1 ounce raw, unsalted cashew nuts

Meal Five

- 4 ounces broiled striped bass
- 12 ounces sautéed red bell peppers

Day 27

Workout

Today will be a cardio workout. You'll be performing your training on the stair climber. I have provided target RPE intervals along with corresponding suggestions for enhancing intensity by varying the resistance and/or step speed.

Minutes	RPE	Notes
3	3	Warm up at low intensity.
2	5	Slightly increase resistance and/or step speed.
1	7	Increase resistance and/or step speed.
1	5	Decrease resistance and/or step speed.
1	8	Increase resistance and/or step speed.
1	5	Decrease resistance and/or step speed.
1	9	Increase resistance and/or step speed.
1	5	Decrease resistance and/or step speed.
1	9	Increase resistance and/or step speed.
1	5	Decrease resistance and/or step speed.
1	9	Increase resistance and/or step speed.
1	5	Decrease resistance and/or step speed.
1	9	Increase resistance and/or step speed.
1	5	Decrease resistance and/or step speed.
1	9	Increase resistance and/or step speed.
1	5	Decrease resistance and/or step speed.
1	9	Increase resistance and/or step speed.
1	5	Decrease resistance and/or step speed.
1	9	Increase resistance and/or step speed.
1	5	Decrease resistance and/or step speed.
1	8	Increase resistance and/or step speed.
1	5	Decrease resistance and/or step speed.
1	7	Increase resistance and/or step speed.
1	5	Decrease resistance and/or step speed.
3	3	Cool down at low intensity.

Menu

Meal One

- 2 slices multigrain bread
- Mushroom and onion omelet (containing 6 egg whites, 1 large portabella mushroom, and 1 small onion)
- 1 tablespoon flaxseed oil
- Coffee or tea

Meal Two

- 1 large pear

Meal Three

- 4 ounces broiled swordfish steak
- 1/4 cup long-grain brown rice (measured uncooked)

Meal Four

- 1 ounce pecans

Meal Five

- 4 ounces broiled filet mignon
- 12 ounces grilled zucchini

Day 28

Workout

Today is an off-day from training—a day to allow your body to recuperate from the intense training that you've done the rest of the week. Try to avoid any strenuous activities. If desired, you can do some light cardio such as walking. Better yet, now that you've completed the exercise portion of the program, treat yourself to a special event!

Menu

Meal One

- Tex-Mex omelet (containing 6 egg whites and chopped onion, tomato, green pepper, and jalapeno pepper)
- 1 tablespoon flaxseed oil
- Coffee or tea

Meal Two

- 1 ounce raw, unsalted peanuts

Meal Three

- Kidney bean salad (containing 4 ounces kidney beans, lettuce, tomato, and cucumber with light vinaigrette dressing)

Meal Four

- 1 large nectarine

Meal Five

- 4 ounces broiled buffalo steak
- 12 ounces asparagus

6

Lifting and Cardio

In chapter 1, I outlined the basic protocol for the exercise portion of my shapeover program. Here I'd like to focus on specific techniques and concepts that, when properly understood and applied, will improve your results on the program immeasurably. We'll cover the importance of warming up, the reasoning behind always using proper form, the benefits of developing a mind-to-muscle connection, the facts on when is the best time to train, the realities of dealing with missed workouts, and the body-firming effects of a specialized technique called isotension. As I like to say, body sculpting is both a science and an art, and attention to the nuances of both of these aspects is paramount to achieving your ideal physique.

Warm Up

Before resistance training, it is important to perform a brief, general warm-up. The general warm-up prepares your body for the rigors of intense exercise by increasing range of motion, improving muscular responsiveness, speeding up recovery, and diminishing the possibility of serious injury. Improper warm-up is one of the biggest reasons people get injured during training.

The preferred method for the general warm-up is to perform a period of light cardiovascular exercise. The objective here is to elevate your core temperature and increase arteriovenous circulation. There is a direct correlation between muscle temperature and exercise performance; when a muscle is warm, it is able to achieve a better contraction. As a rule, the higher a muscle's temperature (within a safe physiologic range), the better its contractility. And because better contractility translates into better force production, you'll ultimately achieve better muscular development.

What's more, an elevated core temperature diminishes a joint's resistance to flow (viscosity). This is accomplished via the uptake of synovial fluid, which enters the joint and provides it with lubrication. The net effect is an increase in range of motion and improved joint-related resiliency.

It really doesn't matter what activity you choose for the general warm-up: stationary bike, stair climber, treadmill, jump rope, etc.—all will accomplish the objective just fine. The activity should be performed at a relatively low level of intensity (approximately a 3 on the RPE scale), continuing for about five or ten minutes or until you've broken a light sweat. Should you begin to feel tired or out of breath during the activity, reduce the intensity immediately.

In addition to the general warm-up, it also is beneficial to perform a specific warm-up. The specific warm-up takes the general warm-up one step further. Not only does it help to raise body temperature, but it also serves to enhance the neuromuscular efficiency of the particular activity. By utilizing exercises that are similar to the actual activities in the workout, the neuromuscular system gets to "rehearse" the movement before it is performed at a high level of intensity. Because of the specificity involved, this is extremely important prior to intense training, and especially during strength/hypertrophy sessions (i.e., the moderate rep days).

The exercises used in a specific warm-up should be as close to the actual movement as possible. If, for instance, you are going to train your chest muscles, some bench presses or push-ups would be ideal. The object is not to fatigue your muscles, but rather to "get a feel" for the particular activity. One or two light sets are all that's needed to achieve desired benefits; then you're ready to go all out!

Proper Form

It never ceases to amaze me how few people actually know the correct way to train. Whenever I walk into a gym, I cringe at some of the mistakes being made. No wonder most people don't get good results from their training endeavors! And don't think it's only the novice lifters I'm referring to; many of the worst offenders have been exercising for years.

Without question, proper form is an essential part of resistance training. It ensures that only the target muscles are used to complete a movement.

There are four main aspects to performing an exercise with "proper" form: efficiency, repetition speed (rep speed), breathing, and range of motion. In order to execute proper form, all four of these aspects must be enlisted. Let's discuss them in detail:

Efficiency   Under all circumstances, a weight should be lifted in the most efficient manner possible, allowing the muscle to contract in line with its fibers. There should be no extraneous body movements, no hesitations, and no jerky, bouncing movements—just one continuous motion, with each rep flowing smoothly into the next.

This process doesn't come naturally. The human body always tries to take the path of least resistance and automatically attempts to lift a weight in the easiest possible fashion—not in a way that maximizes muscular development. Without a clear grasp of proper technique, your secondary muscles will take stress away from your target muscles. Ultimately, structural imbalances are created, resulting in disproportionate development of your physique. Worse, your joints become unduly stressed during exercise performance, heightening the possibility of a training-related injury.

I have furnished detailed descriptions for every exercise in this book. But don't simply memorize these movements; understand their function as well. Know the purpose of each exercise and be aware of the specific muscles that are activated in their performance. As you progress, try to gain insight into the subtleties of exercise biomechanics. The fact is, even minor adjustments in technique can make a big difference in your results.

Rep Speed   Perhaps the biggest form-related mistake is performing repetitions at lightning-like speed. As a rule, you should follow the ABCs of lifting—Always Be in Control. Control is influenced by gravitational force, which, in turn, is dictated by the two phases of a repetition: concentric reps and eccentric reps.

Concentric reps (sometimes called *positives*) involve lifting a weight against the force of gravity. For example, in the seated dumbbell curl (see page 124), this involves flexing your arm from a fully straightened position. During the concentric phase, you shorten the target muscle until a contraction is achieved at the top of the movement. Here, significant exertion is required to complete the lift. Because of the effort involved, a slightly faster pace is acceptable; take approximately one or two seconds to complete this phase.

Alternatively, eccentric reps (sometimes called *negatives*) move with the force of gravity. In the example of the biceps curl, this involves straightening your arm from a fully flexed position. During the eccentric phase, the muscle is lengthened and stretched at the end of the movement. Your focus here should be on resisting the pull of gravity so that momentum does not play a significant role in performance. On average, the negative phase should last twice as long as the positive, taking about three or four seconds to complete.

Try to maintain a rhythm as you train; it helps to establish a training groove, keeping your concentration on the task at hand. Once a rhythmic pulse is established, you will settle into a comfortable training pace. As long as you are in a controlled rhythm, your rep speed will take care of itself.

Because of the buildup of lactic acid, there will be a natural tendency to speed up as you approach the end of a set. Resist this temptation! The last few reps are generally the most worthwhile and you should do whatever you can to push the discomfort from your mind and maintain a steady pace. Remember: the pain is only temporary; the payoff for going all-out is a better body!

Breathing   Although breathing is the most natural thing in the world, it often becomes problematic during lifting. For sure, proper breathing is essential for a safe, effective workout. Fortunately, it is an easy thing to get a handle on once you understand the basics.

Here is the breathing protocol you should follow: Begin by taking a deep breath before starting your set. As you begin the concentric portion of the rep, start to exhale, expelling your breath in an even manner. By the time you contract your target muscle, all of the air should be fully released from your lungs. Then, on the eccentric portion of the movement, inhale as you return the weight to the start position, preparing yourself for the next repetition. Continue breathing in this fashion until your set is completed.

Under no circumstances should you ever hold your breath throughout a lift (a phenomenon known as the Valsava maneuver). Doing so causes a dramatic increase in intra-abdominal blood pressure, which cuts off the blood supply to your brain. Complications such as headaches, dizziness, and fainting are likely to occur. In extreme cases, you can even rupture a blood vessel or tear a retina. Needless to say, the consequences can be dire. Bottom line: even if you breathe incorrectly, it is better than holding your breath.

A good way to regulate breathing patterns is to count your reps out loud. Make sure that you actually say the words; don't just mouth them (if you're in a gym setting, you can whisper them so you don't get strange looks from others!). This will ensure that air passes through your vocal cords and is expelled on the contraction. As long as you continue counting, it's impossible to miss a breath! Moreover, you don't need to think about breathing properly, which frees your mind to focus on the set at hand.

Range of Motion   As a general rule, you should always train a muscle over its full range of motion. In a partial rep, force production is limited to the joint angles used (within about 15 degrees of the angle). Only by working a muscle over its full range will you be able to achieve complete muscular development.

What's more, muscles adapt to the specific range in which they are trained. If limited range movements are used on a continual basis, a loss of flexibility can occur. Over time, the repeated use of partial reps can cause an adaptation in which muscles get used to their shortened position and assume this position as their resting length. Unless corrective measures are taken, the muscles maintain a shortened position, impeding joint-related mobility. Full-range movements, on the other hand, allow the associated joint to approach its stretch capacity. This helps to improve joint mobility, in effect acting as a form of flexibility training.

Mind-to-Muscle Connection

Contrary to what you may believe, lifting weights requires a high degree of mental focus. Your mind plays an important role in the development of your physique and, in order to get the most out of your efforts, it is essential to harness its power. In fact, two women using identical exercise routines will achieve vastly different results depending on their mental approach to training.

What I'm talking about here is developing a *mind-to-muscle connection;* the melding of mind and muscle so that they become one. The mind-to-muscle connection entails visualizing the muscle you are training and feeling that muscle work throughout each repetition. Rather than thinking about where you feel a muscular stimulus, you must think about where you are *supposed* to feel the stimulus.

Establishing a mind-to-muscle connection is beneficial on two levels. First, it ensures that your target muscles perform the majority of work during an exercise. Without a strong mental link, supporting muscles and connective tissue tend to dominate the lift, diminishing your results. Second, it forces you to continually utilize proper form. When you are mentally locked in to a movement, your biomechanics tend to automatically fall into place. This not only helps to improve exercise performance, but it also reduces the possibility of a training-related injury.

Developing a strong mind-to-muscle connection requires consistent practice. From the moment you begin a set, your thoughts should be focused on the muscle that you are training, with all outside distractions purged from your mind. The only thing that matters at this point is the task at hand: stimulating your target muscles to their fullest potential.

As you train, don't just think about moving the weight from point A to point B. Rather, make a concerted effort to visualize your target muscles doing the work, without assistance from supporting muscles. When you reach the contracted phase of the movement, consciously feel the squeeze in your target muscles. And on the eccentric (i.e., negative) action, feel your target muscles lengthening as you return to the start position. Make this practice a ritual and it soon will become habit.

Don't be discouraged if it takes longer to develop a mental link with certain muscles than with others. Generally speaking, it is easier to connect with the muscles of your arms and legs than it is with those of your torso. However, with dedication and patience, you soon will be able to connect with all the muscles in your body, paving the way to better development.

You can enhance your mind-to-muscle connection through the use of a technique called *guided imagery*. With this technique, you visualize the way you want your muscles to appear and then imagine them taking this form as you are training. For instance, when working your triceps, envision yourself with firm, defined arms, devoid of any body fat. As you perform a set of overhead triceps extensions, think of your arms becoming tighter and harder. Make the image as vivid as possible. With each repetition, see yourself getting one step closer to achieving your ultimate goal. By tapping into the power of your subconscious mind, you can take your body to new heights, turning fantasy into reality.

When to Train

There is a growing sentiment that cardio should be performed first thing in the morning on an empty stomach. The theory behind this belief is as follows: A prolonged absence of food brings about a reduction in circulating blood sugar, causing glycogen (stored carbohydrate) levels to fall. With a reduced availability of glycogen, your body tends to rely more on fat—rather than glucose—to fuel your workout. Under ideal conditions, this should result in an increased oxidation of fat during exercise.

But biologic processes don't necessarily take place under ideal conditions. Therefore, although training after an overnight fast might burn a greater percentage of fat calories during exercise, it doesn't necessarily translate into more fat loss. The human body is a very dynamic organism and continually adjusts its use of fat for fuel. This process is governed by a host of factors (including enzyme levels, substrate availability, internal feedback loops, etc.) that can literally change by the moment. Thus, simply looking at the amount of fat burned during exercise is shortsighted. Fat burning must be considered over the course of an entire day—not on an hour-to-hour basis—to have any meaning.

Further, a pre-exercise meal allows you to exercise more intensely (as is required in high-energy interval workouts). In order to perform at a high level, your body needs a ready source of glycogen; deplete your glycogen stores and your performance is bound to suffer. Compounding matters, not everyone functions well first thing in the morning. If you're more of a night owl, chances are that you'll sleepwalk through a morning workout. The net result is that fewer calories are burned during activity—and, perhaps just as significantly, during the postexercise period as well. Remember that following a workout, your body continues to oxidize fat at an accelerated rate via EPOC. And remember that higher-intensity training burns a much greater amount of fat postexercise than lower-intensity training. Impair your ability to train intensely (as can be the case when you abstain from eating) and you'll inevitably impair your ability to burn fat.

What's more, only about half of the fat utilized during aerobic exercise is mobilized from subcutaneous adipose tissue; the balance comes from fat stored intramuscularly (within muscle). The important point here is that intramuscular fat has no bearing on aesthetic appearance; it's the subcutaneous fat that influences body composition. Consequently, the actual fat-burning effects of the strategy are far less than it would appear on the surface.

Finally, studies have shown that eating before exercise actually increases caloric expenditure. This apparently is related to the thermic effect of food (TEF). You see, every time you eat a mixed meal there is a corresponding increase in metabolic rate. When exercise is performed after the consumption of food, metabolism is heightened by about 20 percent over fasting levels. Better yet, these effects are maintained for up to three hours postworkout. And since burning more calories means burning more fat, eating before cardio can have thermogenic effects on exercise.

The bottom line is that, from a results standpoint, you shouldn't go crazy worrying about when to train. Understand that simply increasing the percentage of calories burned from fat doesn't necessarily translate into an improved body composition. Not that there's anything wrong with performing cardio after an overnight fast, but be aware that there are potential drawbacks as well as benefits to this approach.

The best advice is to exercise when you are at your best and when it's convenient. If you are a morning person, go ahead and train early. But if you don't really get going until you've been awake for several hours, by all means train later in the day. All things considered, it really won't make much of a difference in your results.

Skipping a Workout

As I've been preaching throughout this book, dedication and consistency are vital to achieving your fitness goals. It should therefore go without saying that you should resist the temptation to let excuses allow you to miss an exercise session.

Sometimes, however, that's easier said than done. After a bad day at work or a fight with your spouse, going to the gym is probably the last thing you will feel like doing. In these situations, there's a natural tendency to get lazy and say "I'm tired" or "I don't feel like training." Resist this temptation! I can assure you, more often than not, you'll be glad you did. Not only will you be one step closer to getting your body in shape, but you'll feel better afterwards.

Exercise actually acts as a stress reducer. It provides an outlet for your aggressions, allowing you to channel stress and relieve anxiety. Moreover, as you train, the brain begins to secrete *endorphins*—opiatelike chemical messengers that promote the vaunted "exercise high." In fact, studies have shown that exercise is actually as effective as medication in treating mild depression!

That said, sometimes you simply won't be able to exercise on a given day. Sickness, travel, family crises, and other unavoidable issues of daily living will invariably crop up and prevent you from getting in a workout.

If you should miss a workout or two, simply pick up where you left off on the schedule. For instance, say you finished your Day 15 workout on a Wednesday and then had to leave for a business trip on Thursday, without access to a gym on that particular day. No problem. On Friday, perform the workout from Day 16 and continue from there.

One thing you should *not* do is to try making up for your absence by lifting weights on consecutive days. Some people think that a split routine allows you to work out two days in a row because different muscles are being trained on different days. Unfortunately, this isn't the case. Remember, muscles function holistically and there will be interaction between synergists and stabilizers regardless of the split employed. Shortchanging the recuperative process will only serve to set back your progress and impair development.

Although everyone has varying recuperative abilities, a period of at least 48 hours is generally required for adequate recovery between strength training sessions. Hence, the best advice is to stick with training on nonconsecutive days (i.e., Monday, Wednesday, Friday, etc.). As long as you don't allow missing workouts to become a habit, you'll achieve excellent results.

Isotension

As an adjunct to your training routine, it is beneficial to employ a technique called *isotension*. Simply stated, isotension is the contraction of a muscle without the use of an external weight. For instance, if you flex your arm so that your biceps enlarges and hold this position, you are utilizing isotension. The same principle can be applied to any other muscle group. To harden your triceps, simply extend your arms until they are straight. Then, squeeze the triceps as forcefully as possible, feeling them get hard and tight. Hold this contraction for about thirty seconds and then relax. After a short rest of fifteen seconds or so, repeat the process. Spend five minutes or so after each workout using the technique on the muscles you have just trained; in short order, you'll notice a difference in your physique.

Isotension can also be employed in your spare time. If you're standing in line at the supermarket, do some butt squeezes; if you're hanging out on the couch watching TV, tighten your abs. It's a terrific way to make productive use of your downtime.

Because isotension almost exclusively targets your slow-twitch muscle fibers, the potential for overtraining is extremely low. You can use it virtually every day throughout the course of this program without ill effect, helping to enhance both the hardness and endurance of your muscles. What's more, it will improve your muscular control, thereby fostering a better mind-to-muscle connection and, consequently, better exercise performance.

Understanding Spot Reduction

One thing this program will not do is spot reduce fat (nor will any other exercise or diet program, for that matter). The truth is, spot reduction is a physiologic impossibility. Unfortunately, individual exercises can't slim down a specific area of your body—no matter how often or intensely you perform the movement. All the sit-ups in the world won't give you a flat stomach; no amount of leg lifts will directly diminish the size of your thighs. In reality, trying to eradicate your problem areas with targeted movements is literally an exercise in futility.

In order to appreciate why spot reduction doesn't work, it is necessary to understand how fat is synthesized. When calories are consumed in abundance, your body converts the excess nutrients into fat-based compounds called *triglycerides*, which are then stored in cells called *adipocytes*. Adipocytes are pliable storehouses that either shrink or expand to accommodate fatty deposits. They are present in virtually every part of the body. There is a direct correlation between the size of adipocytes and obesity: the larger your adipocytes, the fatter you appear.

When you exercise, triglycerides are broken down into fatty acids, which are then transported via the blood to be used in target tissues for energy. Because fatty acids must travel through the circulatory system—a time-consuming process—it is just as efficient for your body to utilize fat from one area as it is another. In other words, the proximity of fat cells to the working muscles is completely irrelevant from an energy standpoint. Since the body can't preferentially use fat from a particular area, it simply draws from adipocytes in all regions of the body, including the face, trunk, and extremities.

Realize, though, that certain areas are more resistant to fat loss than others. Adipocytes (fat cells) are regulated by receptors that control the storage and release of fat from the cell. Receptors can be likened to doorways; they either allow fat into or out of adipocytes. There are two basic types of fat receptors: alpha receptors and beta receptors. Taking the doorway analogy a step further, alpha receptors are the "entrances" that allow fat into adipocytes for long-term storage, and beta receptors are the "exits" that let fat out of adipocytes to be burned for energy. It has been shown that specific adipocytes—especially the ones in a woman's lower body—have a higher percentage of alpha receptors to beta receptors (as high as 6 to1, by some estimates) and therefore tend to hoard and retain fat.

Because of the effects of estrogen, women get hit with a double whammy. Among its many functions, estrogen is integrally involved in the storage of body fat. Specifically, it exerts a regional influence over lipoprotein lipase—an enzyme that signals the body to store fat. In lower-body adipocytes, estrogen stimulates lipoprotein lipase activity, causing fat to accumulate in this area. Conversely, estrogen has the opposite effect in the upper body, where it actually suppresses the activity of lipoprotein lipase and thereby impedes fat deposition. This site-specific response diverts fat away from the upper body and into the hips and thighs, producing the rounded features normally associated with a feminine physique.

Fortunately, if you follow my 28-Day Shapeover program as directed, you will reduce the amount of fat in your problem areas. It contains the three basic factors that expedite overall fat loss: strength training (which burns calories during and after exercise performance, and increases resting metabolic rate), cardiovascular interval training (which directly burns calories as you perform the activity and increases EPOC), and proper nutrition (which creates a caloric deficit). Although the fat loss won't come exclusively from any given area of the body, you will gradually strip away excess adipose, revealing a lean, hard physique.

28-Day Nutrition Plan

7

I have designed the meal plans to be as simple and straightforward as possible. Everything is laid out so that it is easily applied to daily living within the weekly program charts. However, individual differences and tastes will always play a role in dietary adherence. Accordingly, this chapter provides thorough guidelines for tailoring the diet to your personal needs and preferences. I discuss prescriptions for water intake, a formula for adjusting caloric intake to achieve your goal body weight, ways to substitute foods you like for those you don't, suggestions for manipulating the macronutrient ratio based on your body type, the importance of consuming frequent meals, preferred methods of food preparation, how to spice up your meals in a healthy manner, the effects of alcohol consumption on fat storage, and what to eat after your workouts.

Water

Water is integrally involved in maintaining bodily function. It facilitates cells' ability to send chemical messages to one another, helps to regulate body temperature, and fosters the production and metabolism of energy. Without water, you would die in a matter of days.

In addition, water has many benefits over and above the regulation of basic processes. For one, it acts as a detoxifier, assisting the kidneys in cleansing your body of waste products and impurities. This is especially important when you follow a higher-protein diet. You see, the breakdown of protein results in the production of ammonia, which is then converted to urea. Urea, in turn, must be excreted to avoid negative physiologic complications.

To facilitate the removal of excess urea, your body needs a healthy supply of water. By the wonders of osmotic pressure, water helps to flush the kidneys of urea (and other metabolites, as well), allowing them to be safely eliminated in the urine rather than reabsorbed into the body. As long as water intake is sufficient, an increased protein intake poses no problem to your kidneys, liver, or any other internal organ.

Water also helps to suppress hunger. Although the exact reasons are unclear, it would seem that by filling up your stomach, water activates satiety-inducing stretch receptors. The stretch receptors, in turn, send signals back to the brain indicating a sense of fullness. The end result is that you eat less than you otherwise would. Best of all, these satiety-inducing effects are accomplished without adding any calories to your diet. (Water has no caloric value—no matter how much you consume, it can't increase body fat!)

A common prescription is to drink eight, 8-ounce glasses of water a day—the so-called 8 x 8 rule. However, this formula doesn't take into account individual differences in body size. A good rule of thumb is to take in at least half an ounce of water per pound of goal body weight, spacing out intake throughout the day. Thus, a woman who wants to weigh 120 pounds should consume approximately 60 ounces of water.

On training days, you need to consume additional fluids. As you work out, a large amount of water is lost through your sweat, breath, and urine. If these fluids aren't replenished, your exercise performance is bound to suffer. Thus, you should consume 8 ounces of fluid immediately before your workout and then take small sips of water every fifteen or twenty minutes or so while training, varying the volume based on sweating rate. This will ensure a continued state of hydration, keeping fluid balance intact.

Whenever possible, water should be chilled or served on ice. Cold water is absorbed into the system more quickly than warm water, ensuring a continued state of hydration. Spring water is preferable to that from the tap, as it is generally (although not always) devoid of the pollutants that taint our reservoirs and therefore tends to keep your body free of contaminants.

Caloric Intake Adjustment

Contrary to the claims of certain nutritional gurus, there is no diet that will allow you to eat as much food as you want and still lose weight. The truth is, calories do count and if you want to optimize body composition, you need to get a handle on your portions. Weight loss is governed by the first law of thermodynamics—essentially, if you expend more calories than you consume, you will lose weight. For all intents and purposes, the first law of thermodynamics is immutable: calories in versus calories out ultimately determines whether weight is gained, lost, or maintained.

It is therefore essential that you get a firm hold on how many calories you consume. The meal plans in this book contain approximately 1,400 to 1,500 calories a day. This is generally adequate for a woman whose goal body weight is about 120 pounds. But if your goal is to weigh either more or less than this amount, you need to adjust caloric intake accordingly.

An easy way to estimate how many calories are needed for a given body weight is by using a body-weight multiplier of 12. The body-weight multiplier is based on goal body weight (the amount that you ideally would like to weigh). The formula is simple: just multiply your goal weight by 12 and you'll get a rough idea as to caloric intake. Thus, a woman who wants to weigh 130 pounds would consume roughly 1,560 calories whereas a woman who wants to

Table 7.1   Caloric Intake for Goal Body Weight

Body weight (in pounds)	Caloric intake (per day)
100	1,200
105	1,260
110	1,320
115	1,380
120	1,440
125	1,500
130	1,560
135	1,620
140	1,680
145	1,740
150	1,800

weigh 110 pounds would consume about 1,320 calories. In table 7.1, I've done the math for you, showing the estimated daily caloric intake amounts necessary to achieve various goal body weights.

Understand, though, that the body-weight multiplier formula provides only a crude approximation of daily caloric intake. Many things influence actual caloric requirements, including activity levels, hormonal production, nonexercise activity thermogenesis (NEAT), the thermic effect of food, and various other factors. Thus, you should use the daily caloric intake figure as a starting point from which to work and assess your progress on an ongoing basis. Over time, modifications can be made based on your own personal needs.

If possible, I recommend that you weigh your foods, at least during the beginning stages of your diet. Invest in a digital food scale. They are fairly inexpensive (a good one can be purchased for less than $50) and extremely accurate. Once you've weighed your foods for a while, your idea of portion size will become instinctive. You'll know what a 4-ounce chicken breast looks like; you'll be able to estimate a cup of oatmeal without a measuring cup.

For those who don't want to go to the trouble of weighing foods, here are some tips for eyeballing portion sizes:

- A 4-ounce portion of meat, poultry, or fish is roughly the size of the palm of your hand.

- A 2-ounce portion of pasta, a cup of rice, and a medium yam or piece of fruit equates to approximately the size of your fist.
- An 8-ounce portion of green vegetables takes up about half of a dinner plate.

Food Substitutions

The meal plans in this book are designed to provide significant variety so that you never grow bored with the diet. Based on the law of averages, however, there is a good chance you won't care for some of the foods included in the daily menus. If so, not a problem. Provided you stay within the nutritional protocol, feel free to substitute like foods for like foods (i.e., carbs for carbs, protein for protein, fat for fat) at your discretion. Following are some guidelines for substituting each of the macronutrients.

Carbohydrate   When substituting carbs, stick with those that have a high *nutrient density*. Nutrient density takes into account the amount of vitamins and minerals as well as fiber in a carbohydrate. Not only are nutrient-dense carbs insulin-friendly, but they also supply your body with essential compounds that enhance metabolic function. Many of the vitamins and minerals are used as cofactors that assist the body in fat burning. Others serve as antioxidants that keep cells functioning optimally. And fiber promotes satiety, decreasing the urge to overeat. Examples of nutrient-dense carbs include whole grains, vegetables, and fresh fruits.

Similarly, avoid all processed (i.e., refined) carbs. Processing strips away a food's nutrient density, rendering it an empty calorie that contributes little to cellular function. Consumption of these foods triggers your pancreas to produce large amounts of insulin, turning on fat storage enzymes while shutting off those responsible for fat burning. The net effect is that your prospects of gaining excess body fat are significantly increased.

With respect to grains, adhere to the axiom "think brown" and opt for brown rice, whole-wheat pasta, yams, and multigrain bread over their white counterparts. Brown carbs are slow burning, ensuring that glucose enters circulation in a time-released fashion. Ultimately, insulin remains stable and the potential for fat storage is diminished.

For vegetables, choose greens whenever possible. As opposed to most colored veggies, they are extremely low in calories and can be thought of almost as green water—"freebies" that can be consumed in large amounts without making you fat (a notable exception is green peas, which contain more starch than other greens and thus must be consumed in moderation). A number of other non-green vegtables are also fine, provided they contain a low starch content (e.g., peppers, radishes, cabbage). On the other hand, the consumption of vegetables such as corn and squash need to be controlled because of their higher caloric content (although they still can be integrated into your diet, if desired).

As far as fruits go, avoid anything from a can. Canned fruits are generally sweetened with an additive called high-fructose corn syrup (HFCS). As the name implies, HFCS is a concentrated form of fructose that is super-sweet (fruit itself contains fructose, but in much smaller amounts). Unfortunately, fructose can only be taken up by the liver, which has the capacity to store about 50 grams per day in the form of glycogen. Once liver glycogen is full, the body starts converting fructose into triglycerides—the precursors of body fat—making HFCS one of the worst offenders in promoting unwanted weight gain.

Also, juices are not an acceptable substitute for whole fruits. Juicing tends to remove fiber from a fruit as well as some of its vitamins and minerals. This reduces a fruit's nutrient density, diminishing its metabolic value. Moreover, since liquids require very little digestion, they quickly pass through your gastro-intestinal tract and are rapidly assimilated. This not only increases blood sugar and insulin levels, but it also has less of an effect on satiety. So when it comes to fruit, stick with fresh, whole fruits and pass on the fruit juice (the one exception being during your postexercise meal, as will be explained shortly).

Protein   When substituting proteins, opt for lean sources only. The saturated fat content associated with many protein-based foods renders them poor choices for both your health and your waistline.

If possible, try to buy organically raised livestock. These animals have been allowed to graze in the wild rather than being fattened up on commercial grains. Eating organically results in a leaner cut of meat that contains a healthier profile of essential fat. You'll pay a little more, but it's worth it.

With respect to poultry, only eat the white meat. The dark meat (found primarily in the drumsticks and wings) is extremely fatty, containing much of the fat in saturated form. When buying ground poultry, make sure it doesn't have the skin ground in, as this significantly adds to the saturated fat and caloric content. Also take special care to make sure the ground poultry breast meat; eating a turkey burger made from dark meat is the same as eating a regular hamburger!

As for beef, limit yourself to leaner cuts such as sirloin, flank, filet, and round steaks, which contain only moderate amounts of fat. Anything on the bone or with a lot of marbling should be off-limits. To ensure that red meats are as lean as possible, trim all visible fat before cooking. If you buy lean cuts, most of the fat will be around the edges, so it should be relatively easy to cut most of it out.

Good alternatives to beef and poultry are game meats, which tend to be low in saturated fat and reasonably high in healthy, unsaturated fat. Venison, buffalo, and rabbit make good replacements for beef; pheasant and quail substitute nicely for poultry.

Of all the protein sources, fish is a nutritional home run. White-colored fish are very low in fat, and pink-colored fish are replete in healthy omega-3 fat. When substituting, just make sure you account for the differences in calories. Because of their higher fat content, pink-colored fish are calorically more dense than their white counterparts; so if you substitute pink for white, you need to decrease calories somewhere in the daily plan (either by taking a smaller portion or by paring down a different meal).

For those who are vegetarians or vegans, feel free to substitute beans and soy products for meat-based protein sources. There are now a plethora of soy-based products on the market, including soy milk, soy energy bars, and soy meat. You can even buy soy in powdered or pill form, providing a quick and convenient source of protein anytime, anywhere.

Dairy products can be consumed in limited quantities. Because they are naturally high in saturated fat, though, it's best to choose low-fat dairy alternatives. Stick to products that contain 2 percent fat or less.

Also, about one-quarter of the population is unable to properly digest dairy products (they lack the enzyme responsible for breaking down lactose, the primary dairy sugar). This condition, called lactose intolerance, can cause abdominal bloating, diarrhea, and stomach cramps. If you suffer from this condition, you can either opt for one of the many lactose-free dairy products now on the market or take caplets such as Lactaid or Dairy Ease, which can be chewed or swallowed before you eat a lactose-rich dish.

Fat   The primary sources of fat in the meal plans come from oils and nuts, with lesser amounts found in some of the protein-based foods. These kinds of fat are primarily unsaturated, with an emphasis on omega-9s and omega-3s, and it's important to maintain this approach.

The fat to avoid is saturated fat; it serves no biological purpose and can cause a host of deleterious effects in the body, not the least of which is a predisposition for unwanted weight gain. Saturated fat hardens cell membranes, which desensitizes your cells to external stimuli and inhibits cellular processes. This is particularly damaging to your muscles because it makes them less responsive to insulin, which, in turn, leads to increased fat deposition.

Trans fat (found in margarine, salad dressings, and many baked and canned goods) is even worse. It shares most of the detrimental effects of saturated fat and more. Because trans fat retains some of the characteristics of unsaturated fat (it is made from unsaturated fat), it competes with the healthy omega-3 and omega-6 fat for entry into cells. Ultimately, this impairs your body's ability to use essential fat for cellular functions, leading to a host of negative complications.

If desired, you can use alternative oils such as canola and hemp in place of the suggested oils (try to avoid corn oil; it has a disproportionately high omega-6 content, which can interfere with omega-3 assimilation). Butter and lard are not viable substitutes for oil; margarine that contains trans fat should be avoided at all costs. In addition to nuts, oils, and cold-water fish, healthy fat also can be obtained from various seeds (flaxseed is at the top of the list, followed by sunflower and sesame).

Macronutrient Ratio Adjustment

I have designed the meal plans to contain approximately 20 percent dietary fat with the remaining calories split roughly equally between protein and carbs (individual meals will vary in their macronutrient profile). For most, this should suffice in providing a healthy mix of nutrients that will aid in building muscle while expediting the loss of body fat.

Realize, though, there is no magic ratio that works best for everyone. Some people do better with a little more carbs, some with a little less. I have found that this is often a function of body type, where endomorphs (voluptuous individuals who gain fat easily) usually do better with somewhat lower carbs whereas ectomorphs (lean, lanky individuals who find it difficult to put on weight) with somewhat higher carbs. But this not a hard-and-fast rule, as many factors dictate a person's individual response. Assess your progress and feel free to adjust this ratio accordingly.

With respect to the macronutrients, only carbs and fat should be manipulated; under no circumstances should you decrease protein intake. Consuming adequate protein (in the range of about one gram of protein per pound of body weight) is essential to achieving your physique goals, and is even more important when you are restricting calories. You see, during stringent dieting, there is a tendency for your body to break down protein stores into glucose so that the brain and other tissues have adequate fuel. Because skeletal muscle is not necessary for sustenance (as opposed to the internal organs and other protein-based tissues), it is the primary bodily tissue to be cannibalized. The only way to counteract this is by consuming extra protein. Keeping protein intake high helps to preserve lean tissue, preventing the negative consequences of muscle wasting.

On a cautionary note, I would advise you to avoid cutting out carbs completely, as many ketogenic diets suggest. Carbs are not the enemy. In fact, if you really want to optimize body composition, it's important to include them in your diet, especially when following a high-energy training program such as the one in this book.

Understand that carbs are essential for exercise. The compounds derived from carbohydrate breakdown are stored as glycogen in your muscles and liver. Glycogen is the primary fuel used to power your muscles during intense workouts. It provides an instant source of energy that can be accessed on demand, enabling you to work out intensely. When glycogen stores are depleted (which is what happens when you go into ketosis), your body has to convert amino acids into glucose (through a process called *gluconeogenesis*) in order to meet short-term energy needs. However, this conversion process is very inefficient and fails to supply adequate fuel for training. Within a short period of time, your stamina begins to wane and you ultimately run out of gas. Only by consuming some carbohydrate will you ensure optimal exercise performance and thereby achieve your ideal body composition.

For best results, try to consume at least some carbohydrate in the form of grains and fruit. Provided you obtain the carbs from nutrient-dense sources, you'll keep your body glycogen stores stocked without spiking blood glucose and insulin levels.

Meal Frequency

Some people ask whether it's really necessary to consume five meals per day, preferring the traditional breakfast, lunch, and dinner. Unfortunately, the answer is an unequivocal, "Yes." Although it requires a little extra effort, both anecdotal evidence and scientific research have shown that people who consume five meals a day are able to stay leaner than those who consume only three. Why is this?

First, when you go without eating for more than a few hours, your body senses deprivation and shifts into a "starvation mode." Part of the starvation response is to decrease resting energy expenditure. In effect, the body slows down its metabolic rate to conserve energy. This is accomplished primarily by decreasing the activity of thyroid hormone, particularly the active form called T3. As a rule, the longer the period in between meals, the greater the decrease in T3 production.

In addition, reduced meal frequency has a negative effect on insulin levels. This causes insulin spikes, which switches on various mechanisms that increase fat storage. The spikes then lead to a crash, where there is a tendency toward hypoglycemia (low blood sugar). Hunger pangs ensue and you invariably end up eating more than you otherwise would, often in the form of refined sweets. This sets up the vicious cycle of overeating and uncontrolled insulin secretions—a surefire path to unwanted weight gain.

Compounding matters, the absence of food causes the stomach to secrete a hormone called ghrelin. Ghrelin is referred to as the "hunger hormone." It exerts its effects by slowing down fat utilization and increasing appetite. Without consistent food consumption, ghrelin levels remain elevated for extended periods of time, increasing the urge to eat.

Frequent meals counteract these negative effects. Blood sugar is better regulated and, because there is an almost constant flow of food into the stomach, the hunger-inducing effects of ghrelin are suppressed, reducing the urge to binge out.

The importance of frequent feedings is even more pronounced when you're trying to lose weight. The reason: preservation of muscle. During periods of caloric restriction, the body catabolizes muscle protein and converts it into glucose for use as an energy source. By increasing meal frequency, you attenuate the rate of muscle tissue breakdown. This allows you to maintain more lean body mass and thereby keep metabolism elevated.

To make the task of eating frequently a little less arduous, it is beneficial to prepare several meals in advance, store them in plastic containers, and reheat them in a microwave on an as-needed basis. This allows you to consolidate preparation, thereby heightening efficiency.

Another alternative is to supplement your basic meals with meal replacement powders (MRPs). These "engineered foods" provide the ultimate in convenience. They are nutritionally balanced, easily transportable, and can be prepared in a matter of minutes. Over the long-term, these factors make them an excellent aid in the pursuit of lasting weight management. In fact, fat-loss programs that use

MRPs are significantly more successful than those that don't. In most cases, you can substitute these meal replacements for either Meal 2 or Meal 4 in the daily menus. Make sure, however, to adjust caloric intake accordingly, if necessary.

You can also opt for one of the many nutritional bars on the market. These bars come in a wide array of different flavors and are often quite tasty (although taste is very subjective!). Like MRPs, they can be substituted for either Meal 2 or Meal 4 in the daily menus. Just make sure to adjust caloric intake accordingly. Be careful, however, about which bars you choose. Some products are nothing more than glorified candy bars, containing high quantities of sugar, HFCS, and/or saturated fat (and even trans fat). Make sure to check the ingredients before you buy and avoid bars that contain additives with buzzwords such as "corn syrup" and "partially hydrogenated," especially if they are listed as one of the first few items.

One final note: Don't be concerned if, at the onset, you find it difficult to eat so frequently. It has been said that any activity done consistently for one month becomes habit and diet is no exception. For some it might take a little longer and for others not quite so long, but if you adhere to the same nutritional protocol on a consistent basis, it will become ingrained into your subconscious. Eventually, eating every few hours will be second nature.

Food Preparation

How you cook your foods has a big effect on their caloric content. The healthiest dishes can become fat-laden depending on how they're prepared. Creamed spinach and Southern-fried chicken are two prime examples of "healthy" foods gone bad.

Preferred methods of cooking include baking, broiling, grilling, roasting, steaming, and microwaving. Almost all your foods should be prepared using one of these methods (you also can consume many foods raw, particularly vegetables and fruits).

Generally speaking, boiling isn't an ideal way to cook because it causes a considerable loss of nutrients. Water-soluble vitamins, in particular, are readily absorbed into boiled water. And unless you drink the water that the food was boiled in, you miss out on these valuable nutrients. A notable exception is whole grains (such as pasta, rice, and hot cereals). As opposed to other food sources, grains maintain most of their nutritional value when boiled.

Poaching is an acceptable alternative to boiling. Because the liquid that you poach in is eaten as part of the dish, all the nutrients are preserved. To minimize preparation time, use as little water as possible.

If you choose to fry, do so at low heat (under 300 °F) and make sure not to overcook. Stick with olive oil or canola oil, which tend to hold up well under heat. Use oil sparingly because all oils are calorically dense. An even better option is to use a nonstick cooking spray that contains one of these oils. These products allow you to apply a fine layer of oil to the pan; enough to prevent sticking without adding many calories to the meal. Do not use an oil containing omega-3 fat (such as flaxseed or hemp). These oils have very low smoke points and exposing them to heat breaks down their delicate double-bond structure, turning them rancid.

Avoid deep-fat frying at all costs. This not only significantly increases the caloric content of a food, but it can also fill it with a host of potential cancer-causing agents. It's positively the worst possible way to cook.

Spices

One of the best ways to improve the taste of your foods is by using spices. Not only can the right spices turn a bland, ordinary dish into a culinary masterpiece, but they can actually have a positive effect on your physique. For example, acidic compounds such as vinegar and lemon juice slow gastric emptying, allowing food to remain in the gut for longer periods of time; capsaicin, the pungent ingredient in hot peppers, has been shown to have thermogenic properties, increasing your body's ability to burn fat and helping to curb appetite; and ginger contains extracts called gingerols that stimulate fat burning and aid in digestion. Some of these compounds are also rich in various vitamins and minerals, including antioxidants that promote cellular health. Other spices that have beneficial properties include paprika, cinnamon, basil, oregano, and garlic. Experiment with different combinations and see what you find palatable.

The one seasoning that should be avoided is salt (i.e., sodium chloride). Because it carries an electrical charge, sodium is considered an electrolyte. In conjunction with potassium, it is responsible for regulating the body's fluid balance; potassium maintains the fluid balance intracellularly (within the cells) while sodium maintains the balance of fluids extracellularly (outside the cells). But although it is an essential nutrient, only minute quantities of sodium are required through dietary means (a mere 500 milligrams is all that's needed to maintain normal biologic function—an amount that equates to about one-quarter of a teaspoon of salt). When too much sodium is ingested, fluid is drawn out of the cells and into the interstitial spaces, causing the body to retain water. You get more than enough sodium from the foods you eat (it is found naturally in most foods)—you don't need any additional amounts.

The bottom line is, except for salt, be liberal with the inclusion of spices in your meals. They will enhance the flavor of foods and may even improve your body composition in the process.

Alcohol

For those aspiring to get as lean as possible, alcohol is detrimental on several different levels. For one, it is calorically dense, containing more than seven calories per gram (as opposed to carbs and protein, which have four). And this doesn't include the addition of mixers, which can significantly increase calorie count. For example, a margarita has 600 calories, a martini 250, and a beer 150—given these amounts, it's easy to see how just a few drinks can really pack on the pounds.

In addition, alcohol tends to promote excessive food consumption. It is associated with longer meal durations and unregulated eating. Thus, rather than displacing calories from whole foods, alcohol supplements them.

Moreover, alcohol impedes your ability to burn fat. It is a toxin in your body and your liver must use a tremendous amount of coenzymes (especially NAD+) in order to flush the waste. Consequently, there are fewer of these coenzymes available to carry out vital metabolic functions, including the breakdown of fat for energy. The net effect is an increased tendency to store fat.

Although it's true that, in moderation, alcohol does have some potentially beneficial effects on cardiovascular health, the negatives outweigh the positives when it comes to looking your best. Hence, I recommend abstaining from all alcoholic beverages, at least during the 28-day period of this program. Going forward, you can include them once a week during your refeed day (see chapter 12 for more details on refeeding your body).

Postworkout Meal

The postworkout period following weight training is extremely important for maximizing muscular development. After an intense lifting session, your body is in a catabolic state. It has spent a good deal of its stored fuels (including glycogen and amino acids) and has sustained damage to its muscle fibers.

Fortunately, this sets up a window of opportunity whereby your body has an increased capacity to use nutrients for rebuilding. By consuming the proper ratio of nutrients during this time, not only do you initiate the rebuilding of damaged tissue and energy reserves, but you do so in a supercompensated fashion that fosters improvements in both body composition and exercise performance.

Because glucose is depleted during training, your muscles and liver are literally starved for carbohydrate. In response, several adaptations take place. For one, GLUT-4 transporters responsible for bringing glucose into muscle cells become much more active. For another, your body stimulates the activity of glycogen synthase—the principal enzyme involved in promoting glycogen storage. The combination of these factors facilitates the rapid uptake of glucose, allowing glycogen to be replenished at an accelerated rate.

What's more, the effects of intense lifting increases your body's protein needs. In the postworkout period, amino acids (the building blocks of protein) are used by muscle tissue to repair damaged fibers. If protein intake is inadequate following training, recuperation is shortchanged and results are compromised.

To take advantage of this window of opportunity, you should consume a combination of protein and carbohydrate. This is one instance where it's beneficial to consume a simple carbohydrate source, preferably in liquid form. "Now wait," you're probably saying, "won't this spike insulin levels?" The answer is yes, but that's actually a good thing here. You see, insulin has both anabolic and anticatabolic functions, helping to increase protein synthesis, decrease protein breakdown, and shuttle glycogen into cells. Better yet, any detrimental effects of elevated insulin are all but negated during this time, with nutrients used for lean tissue purposes rather than fat storage.

As for protein, a fast-acting powder such as whey works best. Because it is rapidly assimilated, whey reaches your muscles quickly, thereby expediting repair. And since your muscles are primed for anabolism, virtually all of the protein will be utilized for rebuilding with little waste. Aim for one-quarter gram of protein per pound of body weight, mixing the powder directly into your postworkout drink.

On resistance training days, I have incorporated the postworkout meal as a smoothie. Ideally, it should be consumed as soon as possible after training. The quicker you feed your body, the more it sops up nutrients and utilizes them for repair. Since blood flow is increased from the exercise bout, the delivery of protein and carbs is enhanced, resulting in greater muscle protein synthesis.

If you don't want to go to the trouble of making a smoothie, you can easily substitute fruit juice supplemented with a scoop of protein powder. Grape and cranberry juices are generally good choices since they have a high ratio of glucose to fructose. If whole foods are preferred, a simple carbohydrate source such as white rice or a baked potato along with a lean protein source such as white-meat poultry is optimal.

8

Arm Exercises

This chapter provides descriptions and illustrations of exercises for the shoulders, biceps, and triceps. Before we delve into the exercises used during the four weeks of this program, let's briefly discuss the anatomy and function of each of these muscles. This will give you a clear understanding of the hows and the whys of exercise kinesiology, providing you with the ability to get the most out of your working muscles. After reviewing muscular anatomy and function, we then look at the performance of each target movement in detail.

Shoulders

The shoulder complex is made up of the deltoids and upper trapezius muscles.

The deltoid (delt, for short), is a triangular-shaped muscle that is comprised of three distinct *heads*, each having a separate function. The anterior (frontal) deltoid flexes the shoulder joint (raises the arm in front of the body). The medial (middle) deltoid abducts the shoulder joint (raises the arm out to the side, away from the body's midline). The posterior (rear) deltoid horizontally extends the shoulder joint (brings the arm across and toward the back of the body). It is important to realize that, although the various heads can be targeted, they can't be completely isolated from one another. The deltoid functions synergistically. Depending on the movement, other heads act as stabilizers, maintaining stability in the shoulder joint.

The trapezius (traps, for short) is a long, triangular muscle that runs down the entire back of the body. It originates at the base of the skull and has numerous attachments along the vertebrae, clavicle, and scapula. Because of its configuration, the traps essentially operates as three different muscles and can be classified into upper, middle, and lower regions. Although all aspects of the traps are involved in shoulder joint movement, it's the upper traps that are most closely associated with the shoulders. The main function of this region is to elevate the scapula, shrugging the shoulders up to the neck.

Dumbbell Shoulder Press

Begin by sitting at the edge of a flat bench. Grasp two dumbbells and bring the weights to shoulder level with your palms facing away from your body. Make sure your lower back remains tight and your posture erect. Slowly press the dumbbells directly upward and in, allowing them to touch together directly over your head. Contract your deltoids and then slowly return the dumbbells along the same arc to the start position.

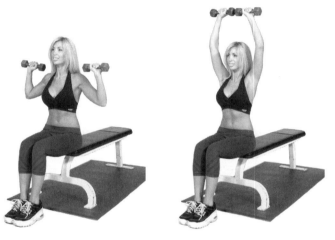

Arnold Press

Begin by sitting at the edge of a flat bench. Grasp two dumbbells and bring the weights to shoulder level with your palms facing toward your body. Make sure your lower back remains tight and your posture erect. Press the dumbbells directly upward, simultaneously rotating your hands so that your palms face forward during the last portion of the movement. Touch the weights together over your head and then slowly return them along the same arc, rotating your hands back to the start position.

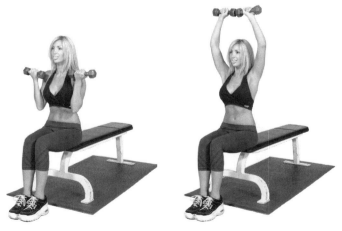

Dumbbell Front Raise

Begin by standing upright with your feet approximately shoulder-width apart. Grasp two dumbbells and bring them in front of your thighs, palms facing your body. Lift the dumbbells forward and up to eye level, keeping palms down throughout the move. Contract your delts and then slowly lower the dumbbells along the same path back to the start position.

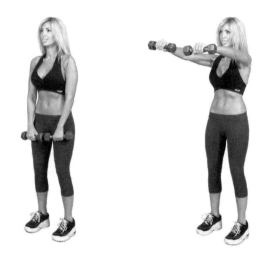

Dumbbell Upright Row

Begin by grasping two dumbbells. Allow your arms to hang down from your shoulders with your palms facing in toward your body. Assume a comfortable stance and keep your knees slightly bent. Slowly raise the dumbbells upward along the line of your body until your upper arms approach shoulder level, keeping your elbows higher than your wrists at all times. Contract your delts and then slowly lower the dumbbells along the same path back to the start position.

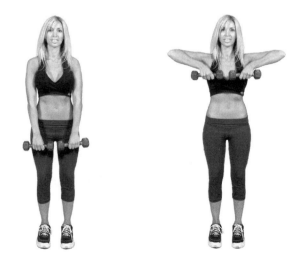

Cable Rope Upright Row

Begin by grasping the ends of a rope that is attached to a low cable pulley apparatus. Allow your arms to hang down from your shoulders and assume a comfortable stance with your knees slightly bent. Slowly pull the rope upward along the line of your body until your upper arms approach shoulder level, keeping your elbows higher than your wrists at all times. Contract your delts and then slowly lower the bar along the same path back to the start position.

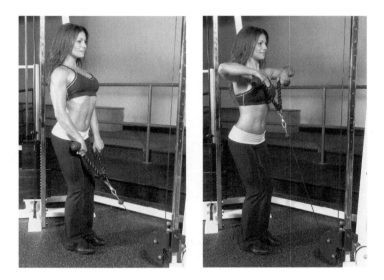

One-Arm Cable Lateral Raise

Begin by grasping a loop handle attached to a low pulley apparatus with your right hand and stand so that your left side is facing the pulley, feet approximately shoulder-width apart. With a slight bend to your elbow, raise the handle across your body, up, and out to the side until it reaches the level of your shoulder. Contract your delts at the top of the movement and then slowly return the handle to the start position. After completing the desired number of reps, repeat the process on your left side.

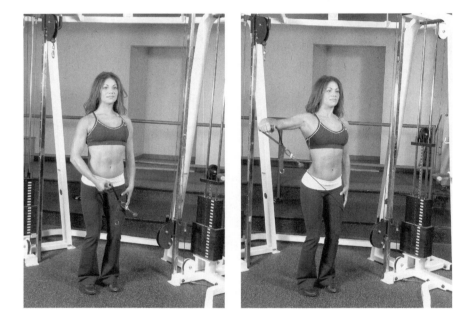

One-Arm Strength Band Lateral Raise

Begin by grasping the loop handle of a strength band with your right hand. Make sure the strength band is secured to a stationary object and stand so that your left side is facing the stationary object (you can stand on the band with your foot, if desired). With a slight bend to your elbow and feet approximately shoulder-width apart, raise the handle across your body, up, and out to the sides until it reaches the level of your shoulder. Contract your delts at the top of the movement and then slowly return the handle to the start position. After completing the desired number of reps, repeat the process on your left side.

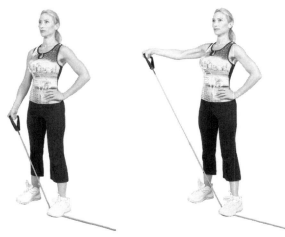

Dumbbell Lateral Raise

Begin by grasping two dumbbells and allow them to hang by your hips. Assume a shoulder-width stance and keep your knees slightly bent. With a slight bend to your elbows, raise the dumbbells up and out to the sides until they reach shoulder level. At the top of the movement, the rear of the dumbbells should be slightly higher than the front (as though you're pouring milk into a cup). Contract your delts then slowly return the weights to the start position.

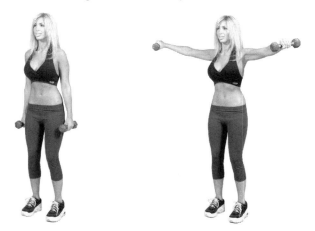

Shoulder Exercises

Kneeling Cable Bent Lateral Raise

Begin by grasping a loop handle attached to a low pulley apparatus with your right hand and assuming an "all-fours" position, stabilizing your torso with your left arm. With a slight bend to your elbow, raise the handle underneath your left arm, across your body, and up and out to the sides until it is parallel to the ground. Contract your delts at the top of the movement and then slowly return the handle back to the start position. After completing the desired number of reps, repeat the process on your left side.

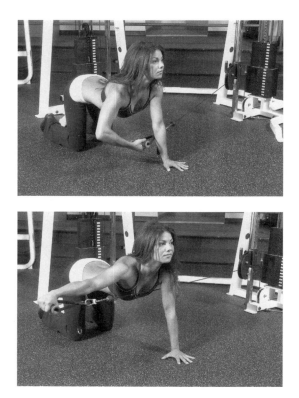

Dumbbell Bent Lateral Raise

Begin by grasping two dumbbells and bend your torso forward so that it is almost parallel to the ground. Assume a shoulder-width stance and allow the dumbbells to hang down in front of your body. With a slight bend to your elbows, raise the dumbbells up and out to the sides until they are approximately parallel to the ground. Contract your rear delts at the top of the movement and then slowly return the weights to the start position.

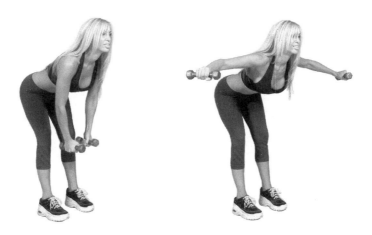

Bench Rear Lateral Raise

Begin by grasping two dumbbells. Lie face down on an incline bench (adjusted to about a 30-degree incline) and allow the dumbbells to hang down in front of your body. With a slight bend to your elbows, raise the dumbbells up and out to the sides until they are approximately parallel to the ground. Contract your rear delts at the top of the movement and then slowly return the weights to the start position.

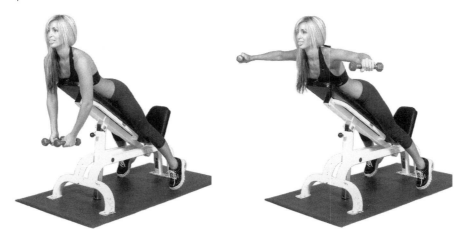

Machine Shoulder Press

Begin by sitting in a shoulder press machine. Grasp the machine handles with your palms facing away from your body. Your elbows should remain back so that they are on roughly the same plane as your torso throughout the move. Slowly press the handles directly upward and over your head, contracting your deltoids at the top of the move. Then, slowly return the handles back to the start position.

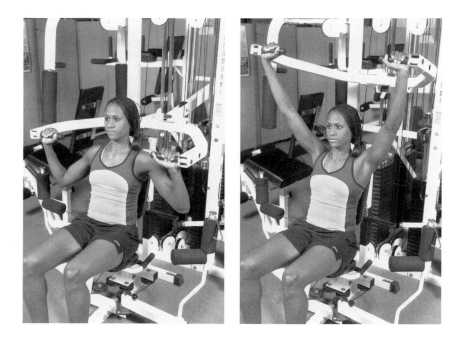

Machine Rear Lateral

Begin by sitting face-forward in a pec deck apparatus. With a slight bend to your elbows, grasp the machine handles with your palms facing one another. Slowly pull the handles back in a semicircular arc as far as comfortably possible, keeping your arms parallel with the ground at all times. Contract your rear delts and then reverse direction, returning the handles back to the start position.

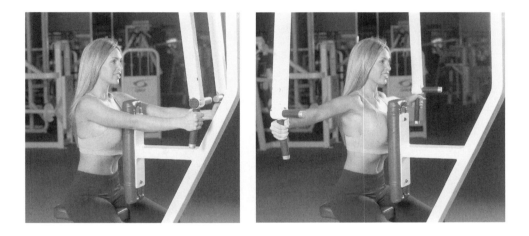

One-Arm Dumbbell Lateral Raise

Begin by grasping a dumbbell in your right hand, and allow it to hang by your hips. Assume a shoulder-width stance and keep your knees slightly bent. With a slight bend to your elbows, raise the dumbbell up and out to the side until it reaches shoulder level. At the top of the movement, the rear of the dumbbell should be slightly higher than the front (as though you're pouring milk into a cup). Contract your right delt then slowly return the dumbbell to the start position. After performing the desired number of repetitions, repeat the process on your left.

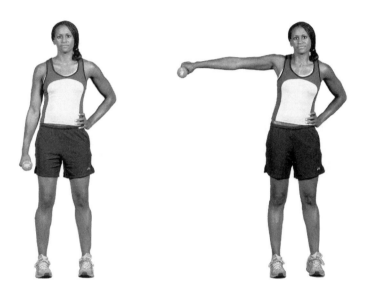

Biceps

The biceps complex is made up of the biceps brachii and the brachialis. The biceps brachii is a fusiform-shaped muscle that has two heads. The short head originates on the coracoid process of the anterior scapula (shoulder blade). The long head originates from the supraglenoid tubercle of the scapula. Both heads attach to the radius (a small bone in the forearm). The biceps has two main functions: to flex (curl) the elbow and supinate the hand (turn the palm up, toward the ceiling). Because the long head crosses the glenohumeral joint, it also has various roles in shoulder function—a fact that allows for additional body sculpting capabilities.

The brachialis originates on the humerus (upper arm bone) and attaches on the corocoid process of the ulna (a small bone in the forearm). It has only one function: to flex the elbow.

Seated Dumbbell Curl

Begin by sitting at the edge of a flat bench. Grasp a pair of dumbbells and allow them to hang at your sides with your hands facing your hips, maintaining a slight bend at the elbows. Press your elbows into your sides and keep them stable throughout the move. Slowly curl the dumbbells up toward your shoulders, supinating your hands so that your palms face your body at the top of the move. Contract your biceps and then slowly reverse direction and return to the start position.

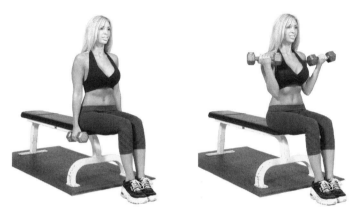

Barbell Drag Curl

Begin by grasping a barbell with a palms-up, shoulder-width grip and allow it to hang in front of your body with a slight bend to your elbows. Assume a comfortable stance and maintain a slight bend to your knees. Keeping your upper arms close to your sides and stable throughout the move, slowly bring your elbows back behind your body, curling the bar along the line of your torso up toward your shoulders. Contract your biceps and then slowly reverse direction and return to the start position.

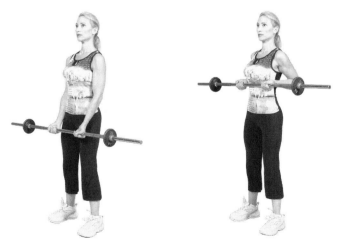

Dumbbell Drag Curl

Begin by grasping two dumbbells and hold them at your sides with a slight bend to your elbows and palms facing away from your body. Assume a comfortable stance and maintain a slight bend to your knees. Keeping your upper arms close to your sides and stable throughout the move, slowly bring your elbows back behind your body, curling the dumbbells along the line of your torso up toward your shoulders. Contract your biceps and then slowly reverse direction and return to the start position.

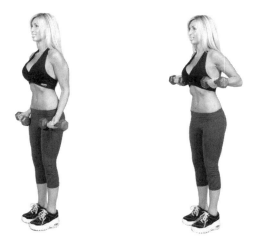

Dumbbell Incline Curl

Begin by lying back on a 45-degree incline bench. Grasp two dumbbells and allow the weights to hang by your hips with a slight bend to your elbows and your palms facing your sides. Keeping your upper arms stable, slowly curl the dumbbells up toward your shoulders, supinating your hands so that your palms face your body at the top of the move. Make sure your elbows stay back throughout the movement. Contract your biceps, then slowly return the weights to the start position.

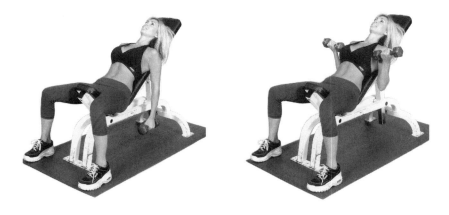

Dumbbell Hammer Curl

Begin by grasping a pair of dumbbells and allow them to hang at your sides with a slight bend to your elbows and your palms facing each other. Assume a comfortable stance with a slight bend to your knees and press your elbows into your sides, keeping them stable throughout the move. Slowly curl the dumbbells up toward your shoulders and contract your biceps at the top of the move. Then, slowly reverse direction and return to the start position.

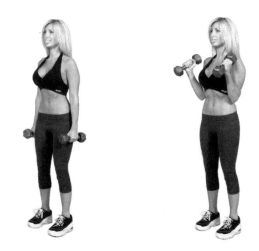

EZ Curl

Begin by grasping an EZ curl bar with a palms-up, shoulder-width grip. Maintain a slight bend to your knees and press your elbows into your sides, keeping them stable throughout the move. Keeping your back straight and tight, slowly curl the bar up toward your shoulders and contract your biceps at the top of the move. Then, slowly reverse direction and return to the start position.

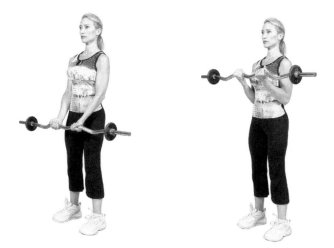

Cable Rope Hammer Curl

Begin by grasping both ends of a rope that is attached to a low cable pulley. Bring your arms to your sides with your palms facing each other. Assume a comfortable stance with a slight bend to your knees and press your elbows into your sides, keeping them stable throughout the move. Slowly curl the rope up toward your shoulders and contract your biceps at the top of the move. Then, slowly reverse direction and return to the start position.

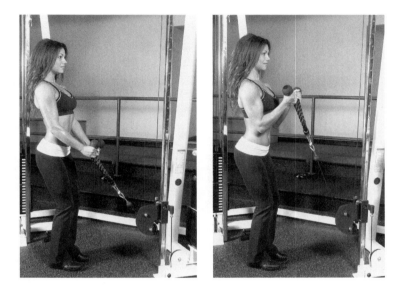

One-Arm Cable Rope Hammer Curl

Begin by grasping the end of a rope that is attached to a low cable pulley with your right hand. Bring your right arm to your side with your right palm facing your torso. Assume a comfortable stance with a slight bend to your knees and keep your right upper arm stable throughout the move. Slowly curl the rope up toward your shoulders and contract your right biceps at the top of the move. Then, slowly reverse direction and return to the start position. After completing the desired number of reps, repeat the process on your left.

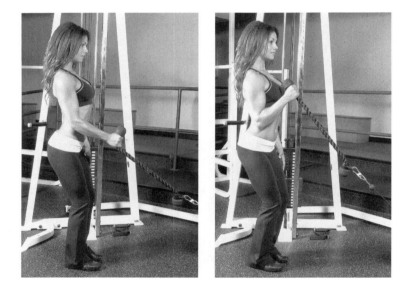

One-Arm Cable Curl

Begin by grasping a loop handle attached to a low pulley apparatus. Keep your palm facing the floor and maintain a slight bend to your knees. Press your right elbow into your right side and extend it downward, just short of locking straight. Keeping your right arm stable throughout the move, slowly curl the handle up toward your shoulders, supinating your hand so that your palm faces up at the top of the move. Contract your right biceps, then slowly reverse direction and return to the start position. After completing the desired number of reps, repeat the process on your left.

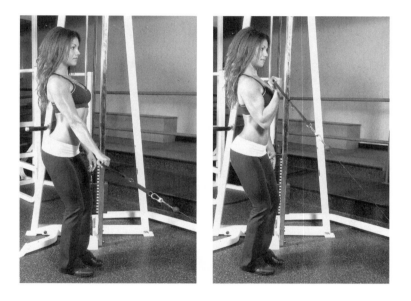

Machine Preacher Curl

Begin by sitting in a preacher curl machine and grasp the handles of the unit. Place your elbows on the pad with your torso erect. Keeping your upper arms pressed to the pad, slowly curl the handles upward toward your shoulders. Contract your biceps and then slowly return the weights to the start position.

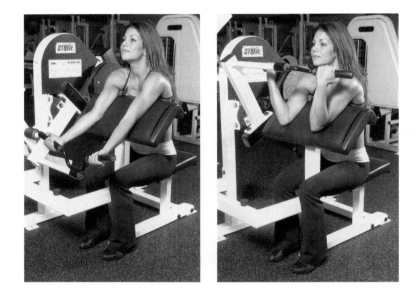

One-Arm Strength Band Curl

Begin by grasping the loop handle of a strength band with your right hand. Make sure the strength band is secured to a stationary object and stand so that you are facing the stationary object (you can stand on the band with your foot, if desired). With your palm facing up and maintaining a slight bend to your knees, press your right elbow into your right side. Keeping your arm stable throughout the move, slowly curl the handle up toward your shoulders and contract your biceps at the top of the move. Then, slowly reverse direction and return to the start position. After completing the desired number of reps, repeat the process on your left.

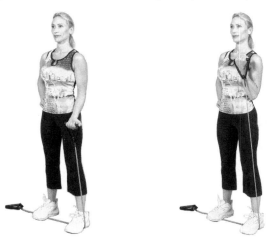

One-Arm Dumbbell Bench Preacher Curl

Begin by grasping a dumbbell with your right hand. Place the upper portion of your right arm on an incline bench and allow your right forearm to extend just short of locking out the elbow. Keeping your upper arm pressed to the bench, slowly curl the dumbbell upward toward your shoulders. Contract your biceps and then slowly return the weight to the start position. After completing the desired number of reps, repeat the process on your left.

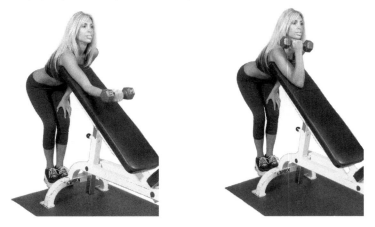

Dumbbell Concentration Curl

Begin by sitting at the edge of a flat bench with your legs wide apart. Grasp a dumbbell in your right hand and brace the upper portion of your right arm on the inside of your right knee. Straighten your right arm so that it hangs down near the floor, maintaining a slight bend at the start of the move. Slowly curl the weight up and across your body, contracting your biceps at the top of the move. Then, slowly reverse direction and return to the start position. After completing the desired number of reps, repeat the process on your left.

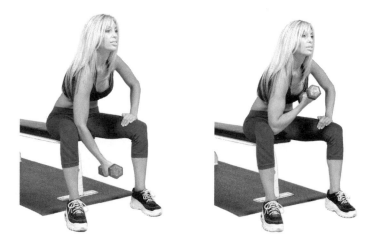

Prone Incline Curl

Begin by lying face down on a 45-degree incline bench. Grasp two dumbbells and allow the weights to hang straight down from your shoulders. Maintain a slight bend to your elbows with your palms facing away from your body and keep your feet on the floor. Slowly curl the dumbbells upward toward your shoulders, keeping your upper arms stable throughout the movement. Contract your biceps and then slowly return the weights to the start position.

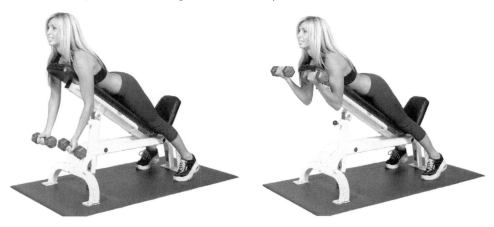

Barbell Preacher Curl

Begin by grasping a barbell with a palms up, shoulder-width grip. Place the upper portion of your arms on a preacher pad and, maintaining an erect posture, allow your elbows to extend just short of locking out. Keeping your upper arms pressed to the pad, slowly curl the bar up toward your shoulders. Contract your biceps and then slowly return the bar to the start position.

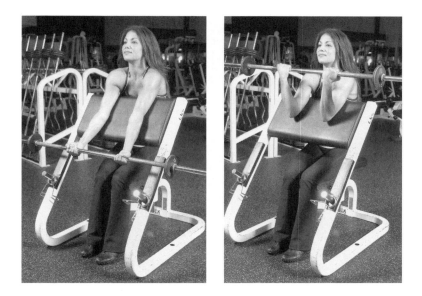

One-Arm Strength Band Hammer Curl

Begin by grasping a strength band attached to a low stationary object (you can secure it with your foot, if desired) at a point just below the loop handle. Bring your right arm to your side with your right palm facing your torso. Assume a comfortable stance with a slight bend to your knees and keep your right upper arm stable throughout the move. Slowly curl the band up toward your shoulders and contract your right biceps at the top of the move. Then, slowly reverse direction and return to the start position. After completing the desired number of reps, repeat the process on your left.

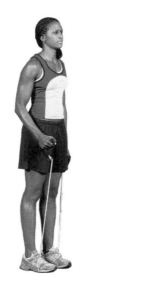 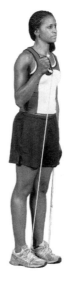

Triceps

The triceps complex is comprised of the triceps brachii.

The triceps brachii is comprised of three distinct heads, each joining to form a common tendon that attaches to the ulna (one of the bones in the forearm) but having separate points of origin. The lateral head originates on the outer portion of the humerus (upper arm bone), and the medial head originates on the middle portion of the humerus (it lies deep and between the other two heads and thus is mostly hidden from direct view); neither of these heads cross the shoulder joint. The long head originates at the scapula (shoulder blade), just inferior to the head of the humerus at the shoulder joint. All three heads of the triceps function to extend the elbow. Because the long head crosses the glenohumeral joint, it also is involved in various movements relating to the shoulder.

Triceps Exercises

Cable Rope Pressdown

Begin by grasping the ends of a rope that is attached to a high pulley apparatus with an overhand grip. Assume a shoulder-width stance with your knees slightly bent and your torso angled slightly forward. Bend your arms so that your elbows form a 90-degree angle. Keeping your elbows in at your sides, slowly straighten your arms. Contract your triceps and then reverse direction and return to the start position.

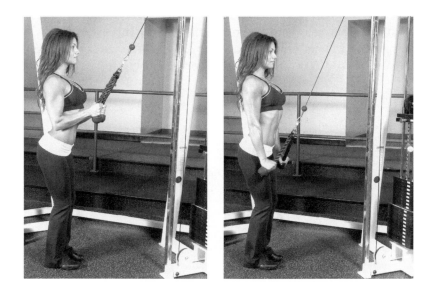

Strength Band Pressdown

Begin by grasping the loop handles of a strength band that is secured to a stationary object. Assume a shoulder-width stance with your knees slightly bent and your torso angled slightly forward. With an overhand grip, bend your arms so that your elbows form a 90-degree angle and your palms face one another. Keeping your elbows in at your sides, slowly straighten your arms and turn your hands so that your palms face down. Contract your triceps and then reverse direction and return to the start position.

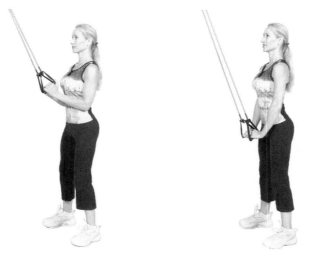

Dumbbell Triceps Kickback

Begin by standing with your body bent forward so that it is virtually parallel to the ground. Grasp a dumbbell with your right hand and press your right arm against your side with your elbow bent at a 90-degree angle. With your palm facing your body, raise the weight by straightening your arm until it is parallel to the floor. Then, reverse direction and return the weight to the start position. After finishing the desired number of repetitions, repeat the process on your left.

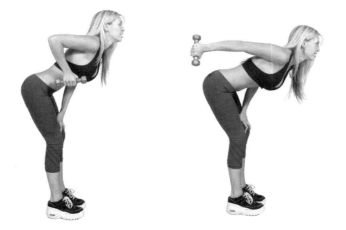

Cable Triceps Kickback

Begin by standing in front of a low cable pulley apparatus with your body bent forward so that it is roughly parallel to the ground. Grasp a loop handle attached to the low pulley with your right hand and press your right arm against your side with your right elbow bent at a 90-degree angle. With your palm facing your body, raise the handle by straightening your arm until it is parallel to the floor. Then, reverse direction and return the weight to the start position. After finishing the desired number of repetitions, repeat the process on your left.

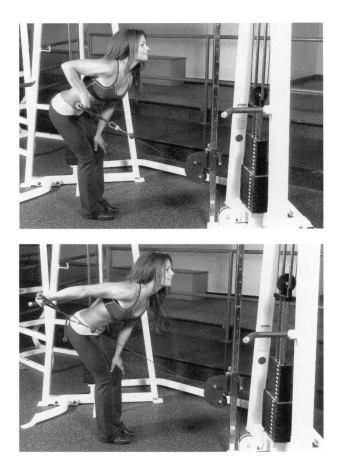

One-Arm Cable Reverse Pressdown

Begin by grasping a loop handle that is attached to a high pulley apparatus with your right hand, palm facing up. Assume a shoulder-width stance with your knees slightly bent and your torso angled slightly forward. Bend your arm so that your elbow forms a 90-degree angle. Keeping your elbow in at your side, slowly straighten your right arm. Contract your triceps and then reverse direction and return to the start position. After performing the desired number of repetitions, repeat the process on your left.

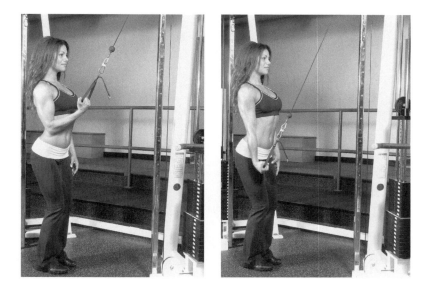

Triceps Exercises

One-Arm Strength Band Reverse Pressdown

Begin by grasping the loop handle of a strength band with your right hand, palm facing up. Make sure the strength band is secured to a high stationary object and face the stationary object. Assume a shoulder-width stance with your knees slightly bent and your torso angled forward. Bend your right arm so that your elbow forms a 90-degree angle. Keeping your elbow in at your right side, slowly straighten your right arm. Contract your triceps and then reverse direction and return to the start position. After performing the desired number of repetitions, repeat the process on your left.

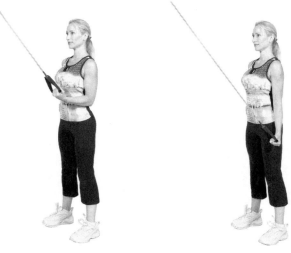

Triceps Dip

Begin by placing your heels on the floor and your hands on the edge of a flat bench or chair, keeping your arms straight and knees slightly bent. Slowly bend your elbows as far as comfortably possible, allowing your butt to descend below the level of the bench. Make sure your elbows stay close to your body throughout the move. Reverse direction and straighten your arms, returning to the start position.

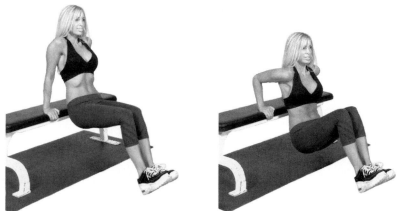

Nosebreaker

Begin by lying on a flat bench with your feet planted firmly on the floor. Grasp an EZ curl bar with your palms facing away from your body and straighten your arms so that the bar is directly over your chest (your arms should be perpendicular to your body). Keeping your elbows in and your arms perpendicular to your body, slowly lower the bar until the bar is just above the level of your forehead (your elbows should be pointed toward the ceiling at the finish of the move). Press the bar back up until it reaches the start position.

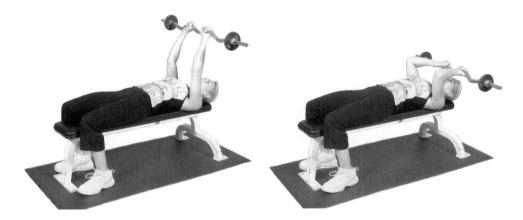

Two-Arm Dumbbell Lying Triceps Extension

Begin by lying on a flat bench with your feet planted firmly on the floor. Grasp a dumbbell in each hand and straighten your arms so that the dumbbells are directly over your chest (your arms should be perpendicular to your body). Keeping your elbows in and immobile, slowly lower the dumbbells until they reach a point just above the level of your forehead (your elbows should be pointed toward the ceiling at the finish of the move). Press the dumbbells back up until they reach the start position.

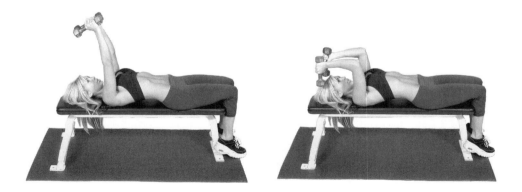

Machine Triceps Extension

Sit in a triceps extension machine and adjust the seat so that your upper arms are aligned with the pads. Grasp the handles with both hands and place your elbows on the pads. Keeping your upper arms perfectly stable and your posture erect, straighten your elbows until they are fully extended. Contract your triceps and then slowly lower the weight along the same path back to the start position.

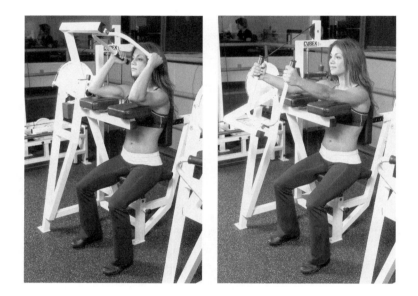

Two-Arm Dumbbell Overhead Triceps Extension

Begin by grasping the stem of a dumbbell with both hands. Bend your elbows and allow the weight to hang down behind your head as far as comfortably possible. Slowly straighten your arms, keeping your elbows back and immobile throughout the move. Contract your triceps and then slowly lower the weight along the same path back to the start position.

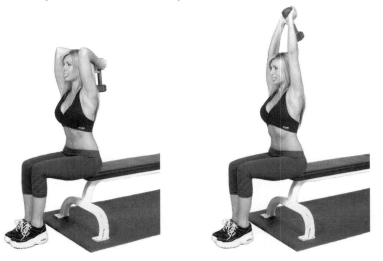

One-Arm Dumbbell Overhead Triceps Extension

Begin by grasping a dumbbell in your right hand with your feet firmly planted on the floor. Bend your elbow and allow the weight to hang down behind your head as far as comfortably possible. Slowly straighten your arm, keeping your elbow back and immobile throughout the move. Contract your triceps and then slowly lower the weight along the same path back to the start position. After you have performed the desired number of reps, repeat the process on your left.

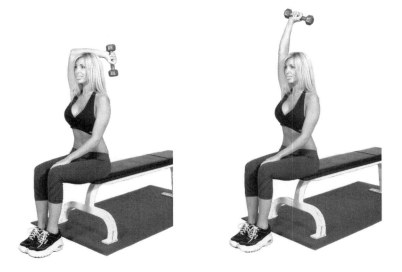

Standing Cable Overhead Rope Triceps Extension

Begin by turning your body away from a low cable pulley apparatus. Bend your torso forward and grasp the ends of a rope attached to the pulley apparatus with your palms facing each other. Keeping your elbows close to your ears, bend your elbows and allow your hands to hang down behind your head as far as comfortably possible. Slowly straighten your arms, keeping your elbows back throughout the move. Contract your triceps and then slowly lower the weight along the same path back to the start position.

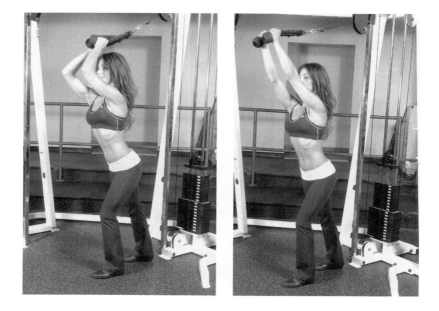

One-Arm Dumbbell Lying Triceps Extension

Begin by lying on a flat bench with your feet planted firmly on the floor or on the bench. Grasp a dumbbell in your right hand and straighten your right arm so that it is perpendicular to your body. Keeping your right elbow immobile, slowly lower the dumbbell until it reaches a point just above the level of your forehead (your right elbow should be pointed toward the ceiling at the finish of the move). Press the dumbbell back up until it reaches the start position. After completing the desired number of reps, repeat the process on your left.

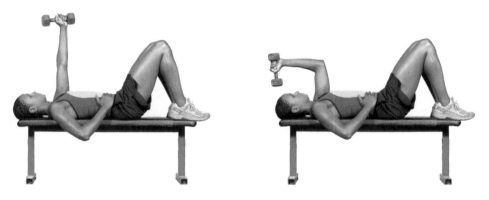

Strength Band Overhead Triceps Extension

Begin by grasping the loop handles of a strength band attached to a low stationary object (you can secure it with your feet, if desired) with both hands, palms facing forward. Keeping your elbows close to your ears, bend your elbows and allow your hands to hang down behind your head as far as comfortably possible. Slowly straighten your arms, keeping your elbows back throughout the move. Contract your triceps and then slowly lower the weight along the same path back to the start position.

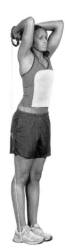
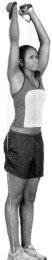

Triceps Exercises

Machine Overhead Triceps Extension

Begin by sitting in an overhead triceps machine. Grasp the bar with your palms facing forward. Bend your elbows and hang your hands behind your head as far as comfortably possible. Your back should remain pressed to the support pad at all times. Slowly straighten your arms, keeping your elbows back and pointed to the ceiling throughout the move. Contract your triceps and then slowly return the bar to the starting position.

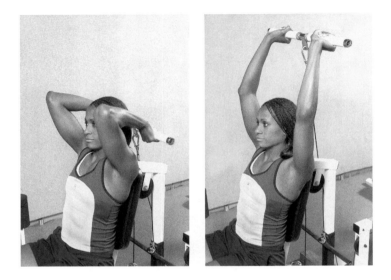

Strength Band Triceps Kickback

Begin by grasping the loop handle of a strength band attached to a low stationary object (you can secure it with your foot, if desired) with your right hand. Bend your torso forward so that it is roughly parallel to the ground and press your right arm against your side with your right elbow bent at approximately a 90-degree angle. With your palm facing your body, raise the handle by straightening your arm until it is parallel to the floor. Then, reverse direction and return the weight to the start position. After finishing the desired number of repetitions, repeat the process on your left.

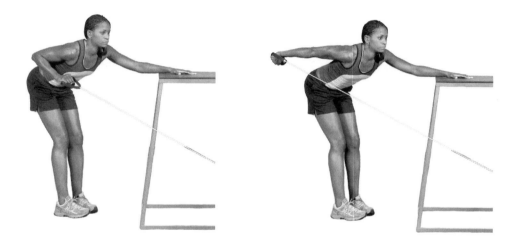

Lower-Body Exercises

9

This chapter provides descriptions and illustrations for exercises for the quadriceps, butt and hamstrings, and calves. Before we delve into the exercises used during the four weeks of this program, let's briefly discuss the anatomy and function of each of these muscles. This will give you a clear understanding of the hows and the whys of exercise kinesiology, providing you with the ability to get the most out of your working muscles. After reviewing muscular anatomy and function, we then look at the performance of each target movement in detail.

Quadriceps

The frontal thighs are primarily comprised of the quadriceps and adductors. Let's take a look at their form and function.

The quadriceps consists of four separate muscles: the rectus femoris, vastus lateralis, vastus medialis, and vastus intermedius. All four of these muscles have an attachment at the quadriceps tendon on the knee. The three vastus muscles originate on the femur (thighbone). The rectus femoris, on the other hand, originates at the hip, making it a two-joint muscle—a fact that enhances its body sculpting capabilities.

The adductors consist of three separate muscles: the adductor brevis, adductor longus, and adductor magnus. These are the primary muscles of the inner thigh, helping not only to tone up the region, but stabilize the lower body and promote an erect posture as well.

Quadriceps Exercises

Barbell Squat

Begin by resting a straight bar high on the back of your neck. Assume a shoulder-width stance with your toes pointing slightly outward, grasping the bar with both hands. Keeping your chin up and shoulders back, slowly lower your body until your thighs are parallel to the ground. Your lower back should be slightly arched and your heels should stay in contact with the floor at all times. When you reach a "seated" position, reverse direction by straightening your legs and return to the start position.

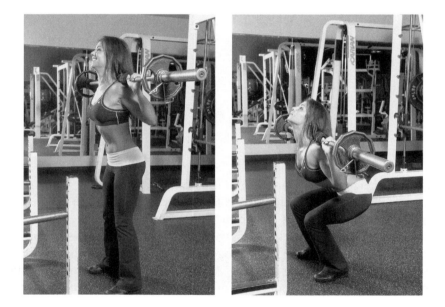

One-Legged Machine Leg Extension

Begin by sitting back in a leg extension machine with your back flat against the back rest. Bend your right knee and place your right instep underneath the roller pad located at the bottom of the machine. Keep your left leg back so that it is off the roller pad. Grasp the machine's handles for support. Slowly bring your right foot upward until it is just short of parallel to the ground. Contract your right quad and then reverse direction, returning to the start position. After performing the desired number of reps, repeat the process on your left.

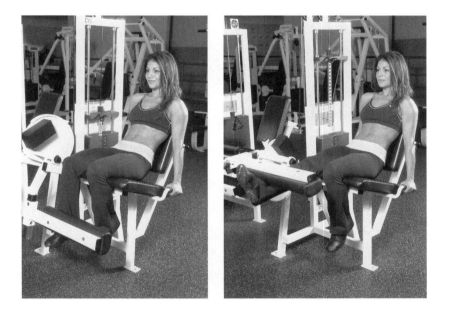

Quadriceps Exercises

Dumbbell Side Lunge

Begin by assuming a stance with feet wider than shoulder-width. Grasp two dumbbells and hold one in front and one in back of your body. Keeping your left leg straight, slowly bend your right knee out to the side until your right thigh is approximately parallel to the floor. Your right foot should be at a 90-degree angle to your left foot and your right knee must remain on the same plane as your right toes. Then, slowly rise back up and repeat this process immediately on your left.

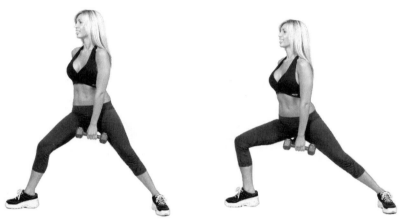

Dumbbell Squat

Begin by grasping two dumbbells and allow your arms to hang down by your sides, palms facing your hips. Assuming a shoulder-width stance, slowly lower your body until your thighs are approximately parallel to the ground. Your lower back should be slightly arched and your heels should stay in contact with the floor at all times. When you reach a "seated" position, reverse direction by straightening your legs and return to the start position.

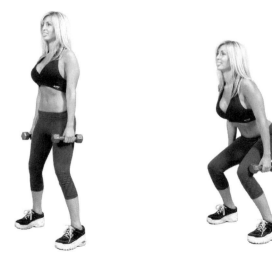

One-Legged Weighted Leg Extension

Begin by sitting on a chair or flat bench and attach an ankle weight to your right ankle. Keep your left foot planted firmly on the floor and grasp the sides of the chair (or bench) for support. With your right knee bent at a 90-degree angle, lift it so that it is a couple inches from the floor. Maintaining an erect torso, slowly lift your right foot upward until it is just short of parallel to the ground. Contract your right quad and then reverse direction, returning to the start position. After performing the desired number of reps, repeat the process on your left.

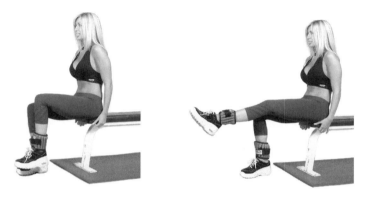

Dumbbell Split-Squat Lunge

Begin by grasping two dumbbells and allow them to hang down by your sides. Take a long stride forward with your right leg and raise your left heel so that your left foot is on its toes. Keeping your shoulders back and chin up, slowly lower your body by flexing your knees and hip, continuing your descent until your left knee is almost in contact with floor. Make sure that your right knee does not go past your toes. Reverse direction by forcibly extending the right hip and knee until you return to the start position. After performing the desired number of reps, repeat the process on your left.

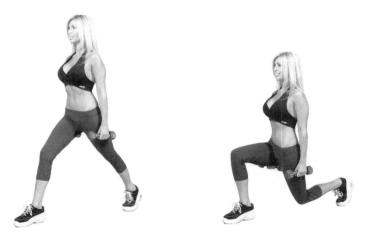

Quadriceps Exercises

Sissy Squat

Begin by taking a shoulder-width stance. Grasp an incline bench with one hand and rise up onto your toes. In one motion, slowly slant your torso back, bend your knees and lower your body downward. Thrust your knees forward as you descend and lean back until your torso is almost parallel to the floor. Do not allow your butt to drop below your torso. Then, reverse direction and rise upward until you reach the starting position.

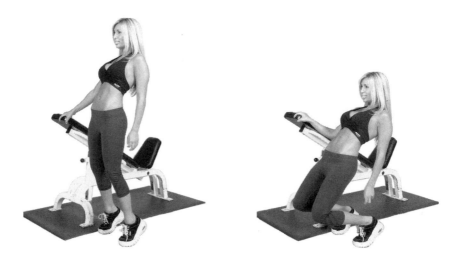

Lying Adductor Raise

Begin by lying down on your right side. Bring your left leg over your right leg, keeping it bent at a 90-degree angle with your left foot planted firmly on the floor. Keeping your right leg straight, slowly raise it as high as possible. Contract your inner thigh and return to the start position. After finishing the desired number of repetitions, turn over and repeat the process on your left. For added intensity, attach leg weights to your ankles.

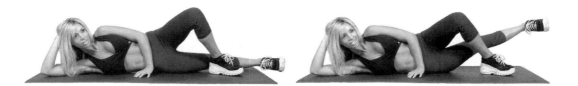

Machine Seated Adduction

Begin by sitting in an adductor machine and place your inner thighs on the restraint pads. Keep your back flat against the back rest and adjust the restraint pads far enough apart so that you feel a stretch in your inner thighs. Slowly force your legs together, contracting your inner thighs as the pads touch one another. Then, reverse direction and return to the start position.

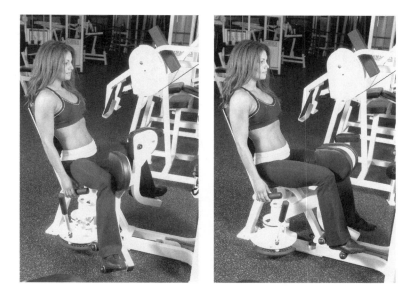

Machine Leg Extension

Begin by sitting in a leg extension machine with your back flat against the back rest. Bend your knees and place your instep underneath the roller pad located at the bottom of the machine. Grasp the machine's handles for support. Slowly bring your feet upward until your legs are just short of parallel to the ground. Contract your quads and then reverse direction, returning to the start position.

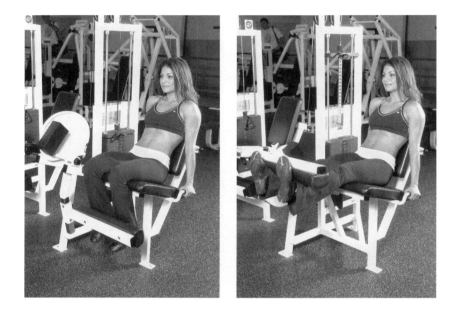

Machine Leg Press

Begin by sitting in a leg press machine, keeping your back pressed firmly against the padded seat. Place your feet on the footplate with a shoulder-width stance. Straighten your legs with your toes angled slightly outward and unlock the carriage release bars located on the sides of the machine. Slowly lower your legs, bringing your knees into your chest. Without bouncing at the bottom, press the weight up in a controlled fashion, stopping just short of locking out your knees. Contract your quads and then return the weight back to the start position.

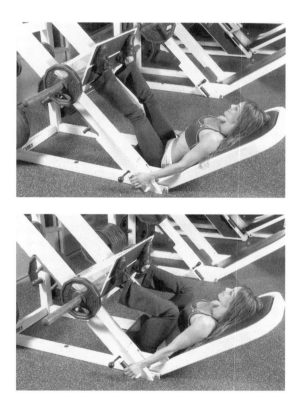

Quadriceps Exercises

Weighted Leg Extension

Begin by sitting on a chair or flat bench and attach ankle weights to both ankles. Keeping your knees bent at a 90-degree angle, raise them a couple inches off the ground and grasp the sides of the chair (or bench) for support. Maintaining an erect posture, slowly lift your feet upward until they are just short of parallel to the ground. Contract your quad muscles and then reverse direction, returning to the start position.

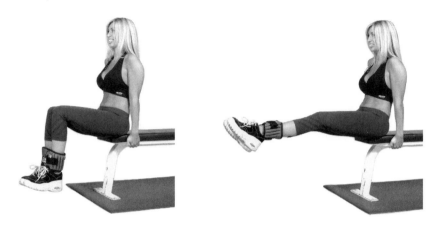

Jump Squat

Begin by standing with your feet shoulder-width apart and place your hands across your chest. Keeping your torso erect with a slight arch to your lower back, slowly bend your knees, sinking into a "seated" position. When your thighs are approximately parallel to the ground, jump into the air as high as possible. Land upright, slightly bending your knees to absorb the shock and, without hesitation, continue directly into the next repetition.

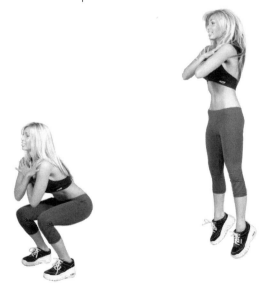

Step Up

Begin by grasping a pair of dumbbells and allow them to hang at your sides. Stand facing the side of a flat bench with your feet shoulder-width apart. Pushing off your right leg, step up with your left foot and follow with your right foot so that both feet are flat on the bench. Step back down in the same order, first with your left foot and then with your right, returning to the start position. Continue with the move for the desired number of repetitions.

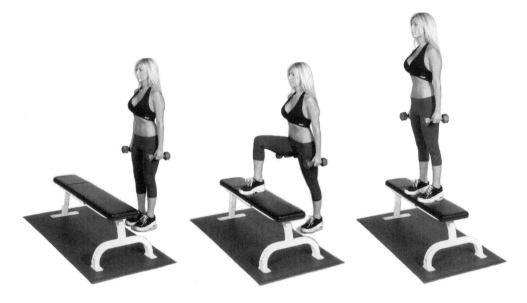

Lying Leg Cross

Lie down with your back on the floor and your feet approximately shoulder-width apart. Your hands should be at your sides and flat on the floor for support. Keeping your left leg on the ground, bring your right leg up and across the midline of your body, allowing it to travel as far to the left as possible. Contract your right inner thigh and return to the start position. After finishing the desired number of repetitions, repeat the process on your left. For added intensity, attach leg weights to your ankles.

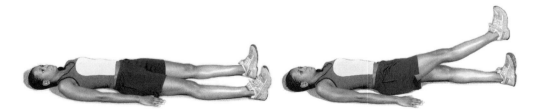

Cable Standing Adductor Raise

Begin by attaching a cuff to a low cable pulley and then securing the cuff to your right ankle. Position yourself so that your right side faces the weight stack and grasp a sturdy portion of the machine for support. Keep your body erect and motionless throughout the move. Slowly pull your right leg toward and across the midline of your body, as far to the left as possible. Contract your right inner thigh muscles and then reverse direction, returning your leg back to the start position. After performing the desired number of reps, repeat the process on your left.

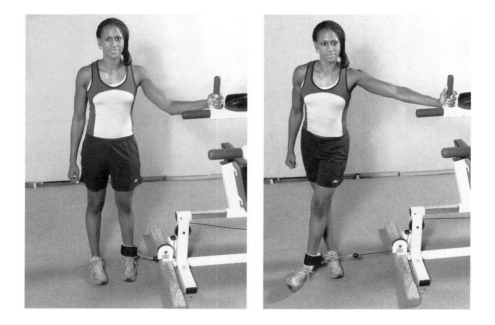

Butt and Hamstrings

The butt and hamstrings are comprised of many individual muscles. Let's take a look at their form and function.

The gluteal group consists of three separate muscles: the gluteus maximus, gluteus medius, and gluteus minimus. The gluteus maximus is the largest of the gluteal muscles, accounting for the majority of muscular mass in the buttocks. Hence, the overall shape of your butt is largely determined by the development of this muscle. Its primary function is to extend the hip joint, allowing you to straighten your torso and bring your leg backward. The gluteus medius and gluteus minimus reside underneath and to the sides of the gluteus maximus. Their primary function is to bring the legs out and to the sides (a movement called abduction). Collectively, these muscles accentuate gluteal definition as well as firming up the hips.

The hamstring complex consists of three separate muscles: the biceps femoris, semitendinosis, and semimembranosus. All three muscles essentially operate in concert with one another, helping both to extend the torso and flex the knee. They reside on the posterior aspect of the legs, originating at the hip and extending all the way down to the back of the knee.

Butt and Hamstrings Exercises

Dumbbell Stiff-Legged Deadlift

Stand with your feet shoulder-width apart. Grasp two dumbbells and let them hang in front of your body, palms facing your thighs. Keeping your knees straight and head up, slowly bend forward at the hips and lower the dumbbells along the line of your body until you feel an intense stretch in your hamstrings. Make sure that you maintain a slight arch in your lower back throughout the move. Then, reverse direction, contracting your glutes as you rise upward to the starting position.

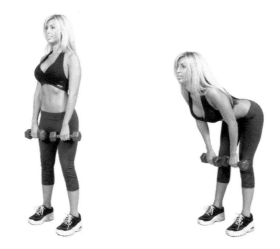

Dumbbell Good Morning

Begin by resting two dumbbells on your shoulders, holding them firmly with your hands. Assume a shoulder-width stance and keep your lower back taut throughout the movement. Keeping your head up, slowly bend forward at the hips until your body is roughly parallel to the floor. In a controlled fashion, slowly reverse direction, contracting your glutes as you raise your body up along the same path back to the start position.

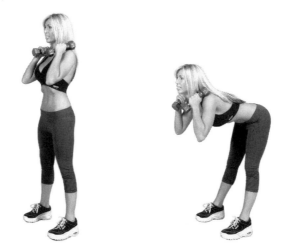

Barbell Good Morning

Begin by resting a barbell across your shoulders, grasping the bar on both sides to maintain balance. Assume a shoulder-width stance and keep your lower back taut throughout the movement. Slowly bend forward at the hips until your body is roughly parallel to the floor. In a controlled fashion, slowly reverse direction, contracting your glutes as you raise your body up along the same path back to the start position.

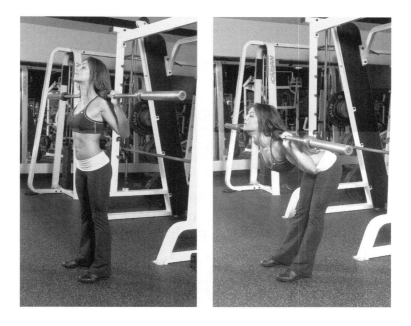

Butt and Hamstrings Exercises

Butt Blaster

Begin by kneeling in a butt blaster machine. Place your forearms on the arm pads and your right foot on the footplate. Keeping your torso immobile, slowly push back your right leg; stop just short of locking your knee. Contract your glutes and then reverse direction, slowly returning to the start position. After finishing the desired number of repetitions, repeat the process on your left.

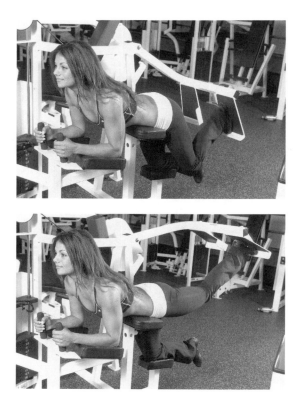

Floor Kick

Begin by assuming an "all-fours" position. Bend your right leg at a 90-degree angle and raise your right knee so that it is a couple of inches from the floor. Keeping the sole of your shoe parallel to the ceiling, slowly raise your leg upward as far as comfortably possible. Contract your glutes and then reverse direction, slowly returning to the start position.

After finishing the desired number of repetitions, repeat the process on your left. For added intensity, attach leg weights to your ankles.

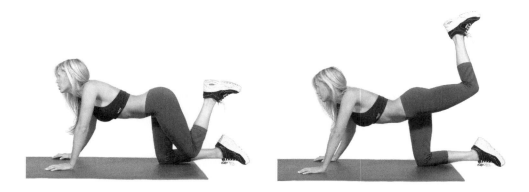

Prone Hip Extension

Begin by lying face down on a flat bench with your lower torso hanging off the end of the bench and your feet just short of touching the floor. Grasp the sides of the bench with both hands to support your body. Slowly raise your feet upward until they are just short of parallel to the ground, contracting your glutes at the top of the move. Then, reverse direction and return your legs to the start position. For added intensity, attach leg weights to your ankles.

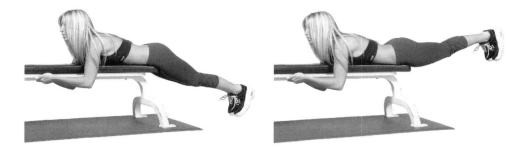

One-Legged Machine Lying Leg Curl

Begin by lying face down on a lying leg curl machine, with your right heel hooked underneath the roller pad. Keeping your thighs pressed against the machine's surface and your back immobile, slowly curl your right foot upward, stopping just short of touching your butt or as far as comfortably possible. Contract your right hamstrings and then reverse direction, returning to the start position. After finishing the desired number of repetitions, repeat the process on your left.

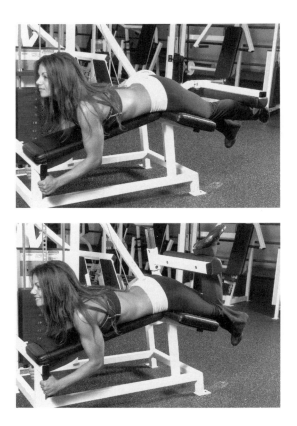

Machine Lying Leg Curl

Begin by lying face down on a lying leg curl machine, with your heels hooked underneath the roller pads. Keeping your thighs pressed to the machine's surface and your back flat, slowly curl your feet upward, stopping just short of touching your butt or as far as comfortably possible. Contract your hamstrings and then reverse direction, returning to the start position.

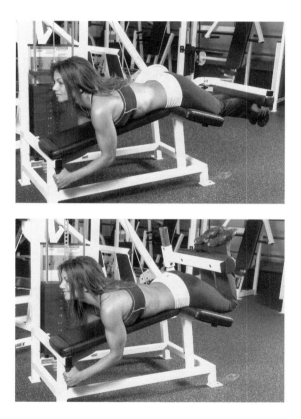

Machine Kneeling Leg Curl

Begin by kneeling in a kneeling leg curl machine, placing your right heel underneath the roller pad. Place your forearms on the restraint pads for support. Keep your back flat and your torso immobile throughout the move. Slowly curl your right foot upward, stopping just short of touching your butt or as far as comfortably possible. Contract your right hamstring and then reverse direction, returning to the start position. After performing the desired number of repetitions, repeat the process on your left.

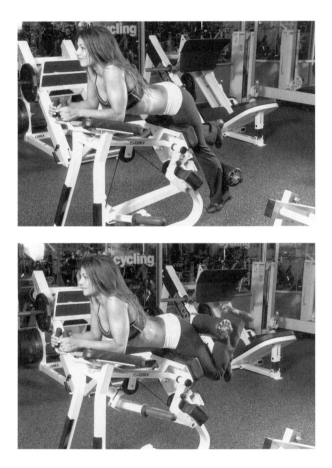

One-Legged Weighted Lying Leg Curl

Begin by lying face down on a flat bench or the floor and attach an ankle weight to your right ankle. Keeping your thighs pressed to the flat surface, slowly curl your right foot upward, stopping just short of touching your butt or as far as comfortably possible. Contract your right hamstring and then reverse direction, returning to the start position. After finishing the desired number of repetitions, repeat the process on your left.

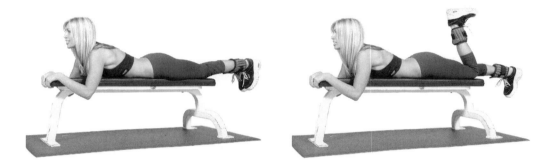

Weighted Lying Leg Curl

Begin by lying face down on a flat bench or the floor and attach ankle weights to both ankles. Keeping your thighs pressed against the flat surface, slowly curl your feet upward, stopping just short of touching your butt or as far as comfortably possible. Contract your hamstrings and then reverse direction, returning to the start position.

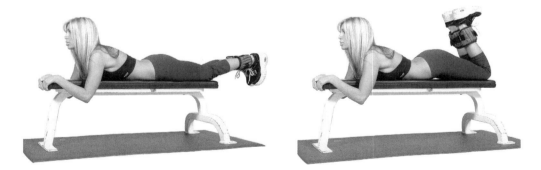

Machine Seated Leg Curl

Begin by sitting in a seated leg curl machine. Keep your back flat against the back rest and place your heels over the roller pads. Lower the leg restraint over your thighs so that they are secure. Slowly press your feet downward as far as comfortably possible, contracting your hamstrings when your knees are fully bent. Then, reverse direction and return to the start position.

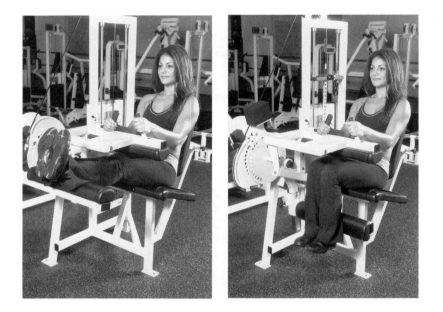

Cable Standing Abductor Raise

Begin by attaching a cuff to a low cable pulley and then securing the cuff to your right ankle. Position yourself so that your left side faces the weight stack and grasp a sturdy portion of the machine for support. Pull your right leg across your body and directly out to the side. Contract your glutes and then slowly return the weight along the same path back to the start position. After finishing the desired number of repetitions, reverse the process and repeat on the left.

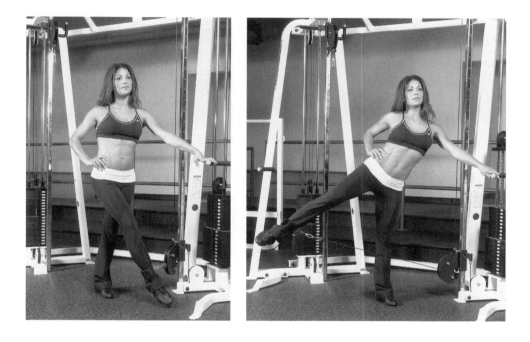

Lying Abductor Raise

Begin by lying on your left side. Bend your left leg at a 90-degree angle and bring your left foot to rest underneath your right knee. Keeping your right leg straight, slowly raise it as high as possible. Contract your glutes and then slowly return along the same path back to the start position. After finishing the desired number of repetitions, repeat the process on your left. For added intensity, attach leg weights to your ankles.

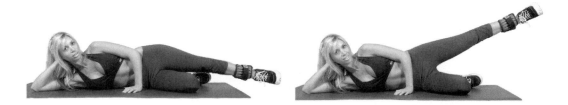

Weighted Standing Abductor Raise

Begin by attaching a leg weight to your right ankle and grasp a stationary object for support. Lift your right leg as high as comfortably possible directly out to the side, rotating your little toe outward at the top of the move. Contract your glutes and then slowly return along the same path back to the start position. After finishing the desired number of repetitions, reverse the process and repeat on the left.

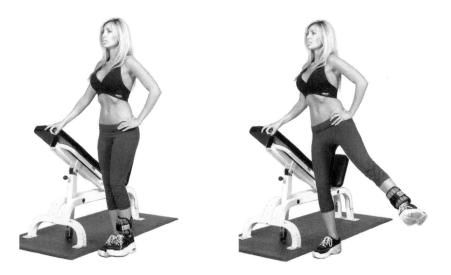

Machine Seated Abduction

Begin by sitting in an abductor machine and place your outer thighs on the restraint pads. Keep your back flat against the back rest and position the restraint pads so that your legs are together. Slowly force your legs apart as far as comfortably possible. Contract your glutes and then reverse direction, returning to the start position.

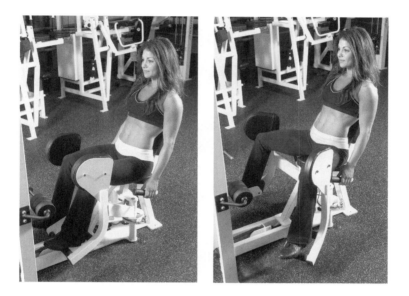

Kneeling Abductor Raise

Begin by kneeling on the ground, assuming an "all-fours" position. Keeping your right leg bent, raise it to the side as high as comfortably possible. Contract your glutes and then slowly return along the same path back to the start position. After finishing the desired number of repetitions, repeat the process on your left. For added intensity, attach leg weights to your ankles.

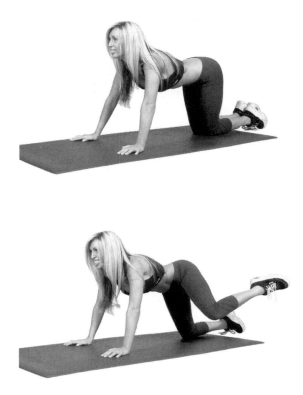

Calves

The calves are comprised of two main muscles: the gastrocnemius and the soleus. Let's take a look at the form and function of these two muscles.

The gasctrocnemius (gastroc, for short) is a diamond-shaped muscle that has two distinct heads. The medial head arises from the posterior side of the femur just above the knee (this head provides most of the diamond shape) and the lateral head arises from the other side of the femur just above the knee. Both heads meld together at a common attachment midway down the tibia and fuse with the Achilles tendon before inserting into the calcaneus bone (the heel). The primary function of the gastroc is plantarflexion (raising and lowering the heel).

The soleus originates at the tibia and fibula and attaches to the Achilles tendon. It is somewhat hidden behind the gastroc but has a much longer muscle belly than the gastroc and therefore contributes greatly to overall calf development. Because it does not cross the knee joint, the soleus can be trained with a great degree of isolation by performing calf exercises with the knees bent.

Machine Standing Calf Raise

Begin by placing your shoulders on the restraint pads of a standing calf machine. Place the balls of your feet on the footplate and drop your heels below your toes. Slowly rise as high as you can onto your toes until your calves are fully flexed. Contract your calves and then slowly reverse direction, returning to the starting position.

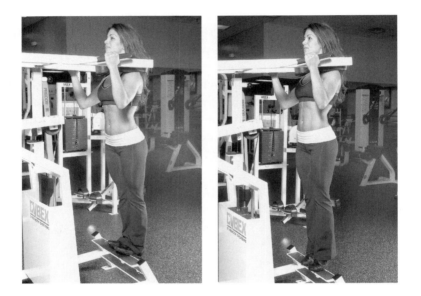

One-Legged Machine Seated Calf Raise

Begin by sitting in a seated calf machine and place the restraint pads tightly across your right thigh, keeping your left leg free from the restraint pad. Place the ball of your right foot on the footplate and drop your right heel as far below your toes as possible. Slowly rise as high as you can onto your right toes until your calves are fully flexed. Contract your calves and then slowly reverse direction, returning to the starting position. After performing the desired number of repetitions, repeat the process on your left.

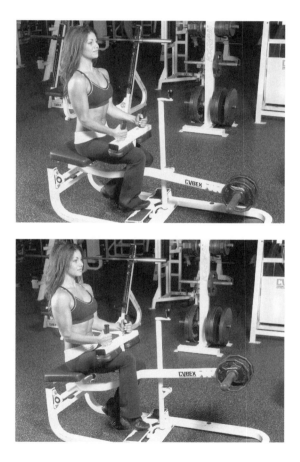

Dumbbell Standing Calf Raise

Begin by standing on a step (or staircase) and allow your heels to drop below your toes. Hold onto a stationary object with one hand and hold a dumbbell in the other hand. Slowly rise as high as you can onto your toes until your calves are fully flexed. Contract your calves and then slowly reverse direction, returning to the starting position.

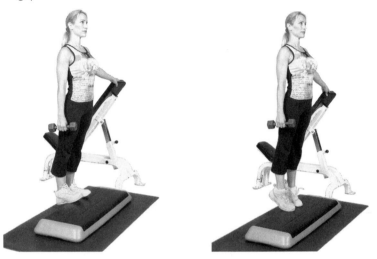

One-Legged Dumbbell Seated Calf Raise

Begin by sitting at the edge of a flat bench with the ball of your right foot on a block of wood or a step. Place a dumbbell on your thigh and hold it in place and drop your right heel as far below your toes as possible. Keeping your left foot back, slowly rise as high as you can onto your right toes until your calves are fully flexed. Contract your calf muscles and then slowly reverse direction, returning to the starting position. After performing the desired number of repetitions, repeat the process on your left.

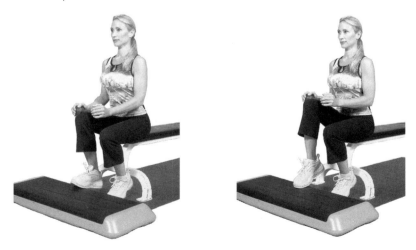

One-Legged Toe Press

Begin by sitting in a leg press machine, pressing your back firmly against the padded seat. Place the ball of your right foot on the bottom of the footplate keeping your right heel off the footplate. Rest your left leg on the floor or in a comfortable position away from the footplate. Straighten your right leg, unlock the carriage release bars, and drop your right heel below your toes. Keeping your right knee stable, slowly press your right toes as high up as you can. Contract your calves and then slowly reverse direction, returning to the starting position. After performing the desired number of repetitions, repeat the process on your left.

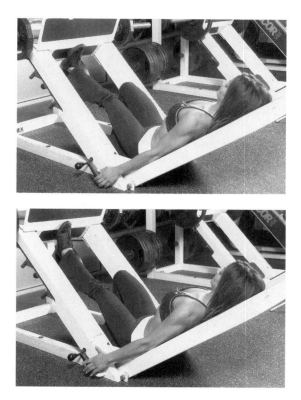

Machine Seated Calf Raise

Begin by sitting in a seated calf machine and place the restraint pads tightly across your thighs. Place the balls of your feet on the footplate and drop your heels as far below your toes as possible. Slowly rise as high as you can onto your toes until your calves are fully flexed. Contract your calves and then slowly reverse direction, returning to the starting position.

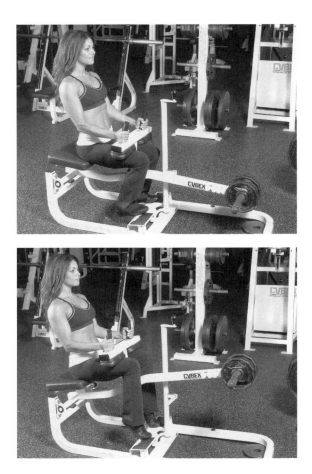

One-Legged Dumbbell Standing Calf Raise

Begin by standing on a step (or staircase) with your right leg and allow your right heel to drop below your toes. Keeping your left leg behind your body, hold onto a stationary object with one hand and hold a dumbbell in the other hand. Slowly rise as high as you can onto your toes until your right calf muscles are fully flexed. Contract your calves and then slowly reverse direction, returning to the starting position. Repeat with your left leg after finishing the desired reps on your right.

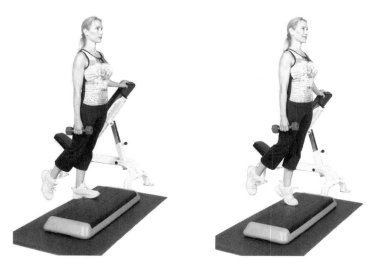

Dumbbell Seated Calf Raise

Begin by sitting at the edge of a flat bench with the balls of your feet on a block of wood or step. Place a dumbbell on your thighs and hold it in place and drop your heels as far below your toes as possible. Slowly rise as high as you can onto your toes until your calves are fully flexed. Contract your calves and then slowly reverse direction, returning to the starting position.

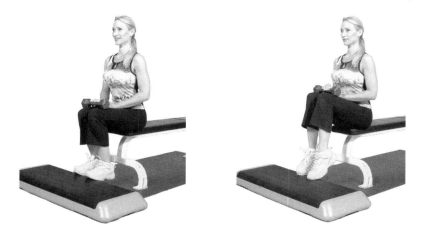

One-Legged Machine Standing Calf Raise

Begin by placing your shoulders on the restraint pads of a standing calf machine. Place the ball of your right foot on the footplate and drop your right heel below your toes. Your left leg should remain comfortably behind your body. Slowly rise as high as you can onto your right toes until your calf muscles are fully flexed. Contract your calves and then slowly reverse direction, returning to the starting position. Repeat with your left leg after finishing the desired reps on your right.

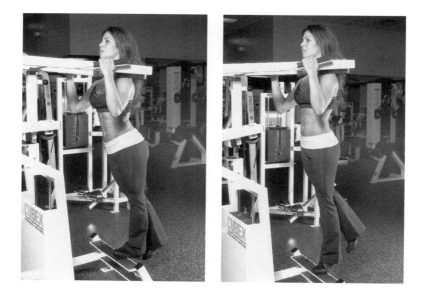

Toe Press

Begin by sitting in a leg press machine, pressing your back firmly against the padded seat. Place the balls of your feet a comfortable distance apart on the bottom of the footplate; keeping your heels off the footplate. Straighten your legs, unlock the carriage release bars, and drop your heels below your toes. Keeping your knees stable, slowly press your toes as high up as you can. Contract your calves and then slowly reverse direction, returning to the starting position.

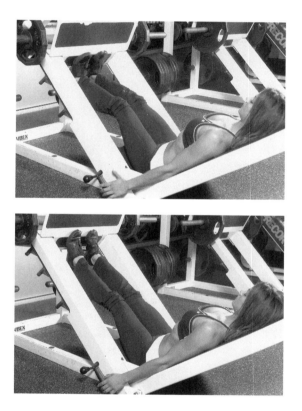

10

Torso Exercises

This chapter provides descriptions and illustrations for exercises for the chest, back, and abdominals. Before we delve into the exercises used during the four weeks of this program, let's briefly discuss the anatomy and function of each of these muscles. This will give you a clear understanding of the hows and the whys of exercise kinesiology, providing you with the ability to get the most out of your working muscles. After reviewing muscular anatomy and function, we then look at the performance of each target movement in detail.

Chest

The chest is comprised of the pectorals (pecs, for short). Let's take a look at their form and function.

The pectoralis major is a large, sunburst-shaped muscle that has two heads. The clavicular head originates on the front of the clavicle (collarbone) and the sternocostal head originates on the manubrium (the top of the sternum) as well as the upper six ribs. Both heads attach to the humerus (upper arm bone) and have similar functions in shoulder joint adduction (bringing the arm across the midline of the body) and medial rotation of the upper arm. Because of their different origins, however, each head also has its own unique function. Namely, the clavicular head helps to flex the shoulder joint whereas the sternocostal head helps to extend it.

The pectoralis minor is a small, straplike muscle. It originates on the third, fourth, and fifth ribs and inserts on the coracoid process of the scapula (shoulder blade). Although its main function is scapular depression, it also assists the pectoralis major by abducting the scapula during various chest movements.

Barbell Incline Press

Begin by lying face up on an incline bench set at approximately 30 to 40 degrees, planting your feet firmly on the floor. Grasp a barbell with a shoulder-width grip and bring it down to the upper aspect of your chest. Press the bar directly over your upper chest, moving it in a straight line into the air. Feel a contraction in your chest muscles at the top of the movement and then slowly reverse direction, returning to the starting position.

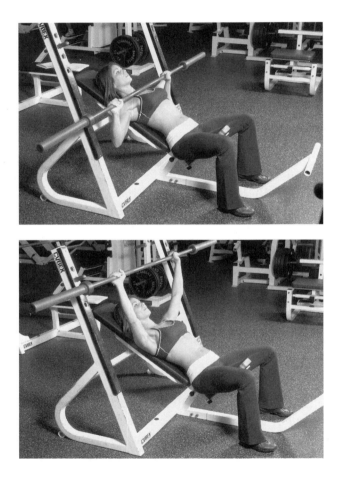

Dumbbell Flat Press

Begin by lying face up on a flat bench with your feet planted firmly on the floor. Grasp two dumbbells and, with your palms facing away from your body, bring your elbows to shoulder level so that they rest just above your armpits. Simultaneously press both dumbbells directly over your chest, moving them in toward each other on the ascent. At the finish of the movement, the sides of the dumbbells should gently touch together. Feel a contraction in your chest muscles at the top of the movement and then slowly reverse direction, returning to the starting position.

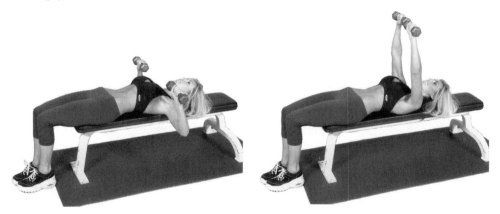

Dumbbell Incline Fly

Begin by lying on an incline bench set at approximately 30 to 40 degrees, planting your feet firmly on the floor. Grasp two dumbbells and bring them out to your sides, maintaining a slight bend to your elbows throughout the move. Your palms should be facing in and toward the ceiling, and your upper arms should be roughly parallel to the level of the bench. Slowly raise the weights upward in a circular motion, as if you were hugging a large tree. Gently touch the weights together at the top of the move and, after feeling a contraction in your chest muscles, slowly return the weights along the same path back to the start position.

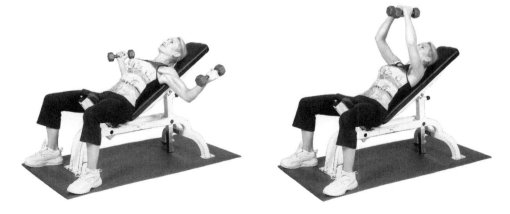

Dumbbell Incline Press

Begin by lying face up on an incline bench, planting your feet firmly on the floor. Grasp two dumbbells and, with your palms facing away from your body, bring them to shoulder level so that they rest just above your armpits. Simultaneously press both dumbbells directly over your chest, moving them in toward each other on the ascent. At the finish of the movement, the sides of the dumbbells should gently touch together. Feel a contraction in your chest muscles and then slowly reverse direction, returning to the starting position.

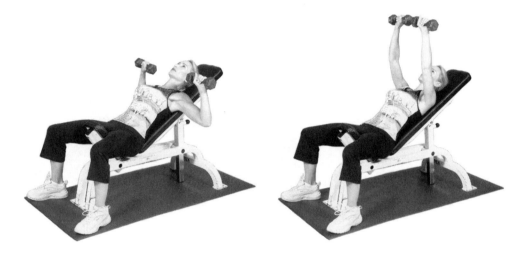

Push-Up

Begin with your hands and toes on the floor. Your torso and legs should remain rigid, keeping your back perfectly straight throughout the move. Bend your arms and slowly lower your body downward, stopping just before your chest touches the ground. Feel a stretch in your chest muscles and then reverse direction, pushing your body up along the same path back to the start position.

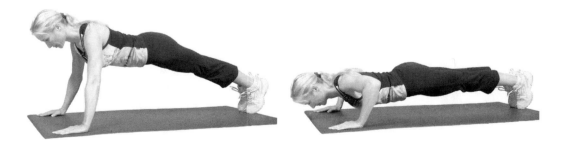

Machine Incline Chest Press

Begin by sitting in a chest press machine with an erect posture, aligning your upper chest with the handles of the machine. Grasp the handles with a shoulder-width grip, keeping your palms facing away from your body. Slowly press the handles forward, stopping just before you fully lock out your elbows. Feel a contraction in your chest muscles at the finish of the movement and then slowly reverse direction, returning to the starting position.

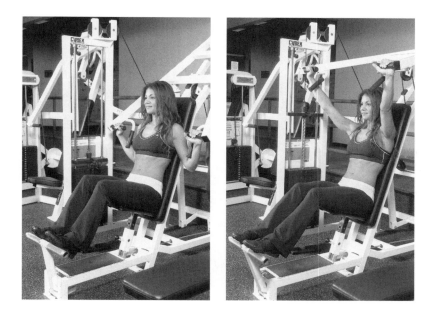

Dumbbell Flat Fly

Begin by lying on a flat bench, planting your feet firmly on the floor. Grasp two dumbbells and bring them out to your sides, maintaining a slight bend to your elbows throughout the move. Your palms should be facing in and toward the ceiling, and your upper arms should be roughly parallel with the level of the bench. Slowly raise the weights upward in a semicircular motion, as if you were hugging a large tree. Gently touch the weights together at the top of the move and, after feeling a contraction in your chest muscles, slowly return the weights along the same path back to the start position.

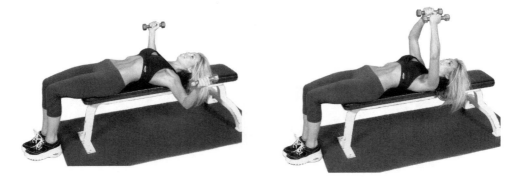

Dumbbell Incline Fly

Begin by lying on an incline bench set at approximately 30 to 40 degrees, planting your feet firmly on the floor. Grasp two dumbbells and bring them out to your sides, maintaining a slight bend to your elbows throughout the move. Your palms should be facing in and toward the ceiling, and your upper arms should be roughly parallel to and at the level of the bench. Slowly raise the weights upward in a circular motion, as if you were hugging a large tree. Gently touch the weights together at the top of the move and, after feeling a contraction in your chest muscles, slowly return the weights along the same path back to the start position.

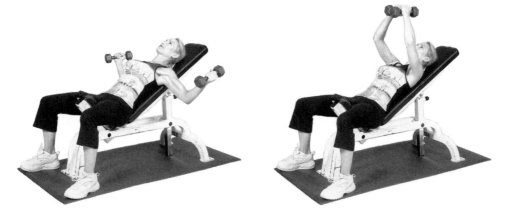

Cable Low Pulley Crossover

Begin by grasping the loop handles of a low pulley apparatus (cable crossover machine). Stand with your feet staggered and your torso bent slightly forward at the waist. Slowly pull both handles up and across your body, creating a semicircular movement with your arms. Bring your hands together at the level of your chest and squeeze your pectoral muscles so that you feel a contraction in the cleavage area. Then, slowly reverse direction, allowing your hands to return along the same path back to the start position.

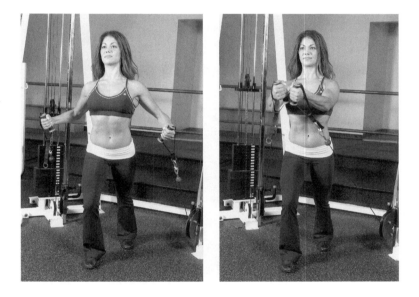

Machine Flat Press

Begin by lying in a chest press machine, aligning your mid chest with the handles on the machine. Grasp the handles with a shoulder-width grip, keeping your palms facing away from your body and your back pressed against the support pad at all times. Slowly press the handles upward, stopping just before you fully lock out your elbows. Feel a contraction in your chest muscles at the finish of the movement and then slowly reverse direction, returning to the starting position.

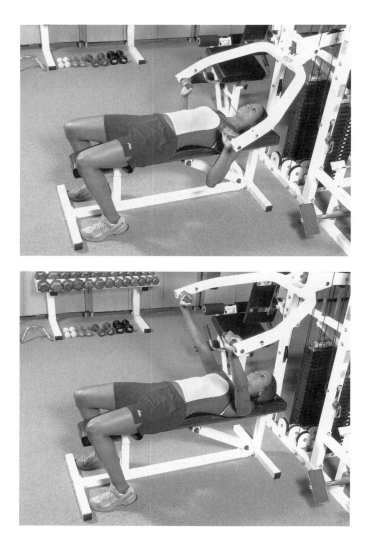

Cable High Pulley Crossover

Begin by grasping the handles of an overhead pulley apparatus (cable crossover machine). Stand with your feet staggered and your torso bent slightly forward at the waist. Your back should remain tight and motionless throughout the move. Slowly pull both handles downward and across your body, creating a semicircular movement. Bring your hands together at the level of your hips and squeeze your chest muscles so that you feel a contraction in the cleavage area. Then, slowly reverse direction, allowing your hands to return along the same path back to the start position.

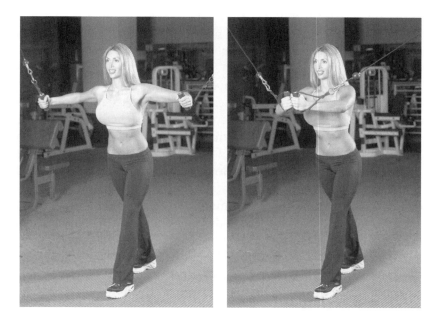

Back

The upper back is the most complex of all muscle groups, comprising many individual muscles. Let's take a look at the most important of these muscles from a body sculpting perspective.

The latissimus dorsi is a broad, flat muscle most often associated with upper back muscularity. It attaches superiorly at the upper portion of the humerus (i.e., upper arm) and distally at multiple points along the vertebrae, hip, ribs, thoracolumbar fascia, and, in some people, the inferior angle of the scapula. Its fibers have several different angles of pull depending on where the origins of the fibers are located, and thus the muscle has multiple functions including to extend the humerus (pull the upper arm backward), adduct the humerus (pull the arms down toward the sides of the body), and medially rotate the humerus (rotate the shoulder so that if the palm of the hand is facing forward, it would be turned toward the body).

The teres major originates at the upper portion of the humerus and attaches distally on the inferior portion of the scapula. Its primary function is to adduct the humerus (pull the arms down toward the sides of the body).

As discussed in chapter 8, the trapezius (traps, for short) is a long, triangular muscle that runs down the entire back of the body. It originates at the base of the skull and has numerous attachments along the vertebrae, clavicle, and scapula. Because the middle fibers run horizontally across and the lower fibers course horizontally upward, these are the primary aspects of the trapezius involved in upper back movements, assisting in adducting and lowering the scapula.

The rhomboids reside in the middle of the upper back and are classified into the rhomboid major and the rhomboid minor. The rhomboid major attaches superiorly at the seventh cervical and first thoracic vertebrae and distally at the medial border of the scapula. The rhomboid minor attaches at the second through fifth thoracic vertebrae and inserts along the medial border of the scapula just above the rhomboid major. These muscles lie deep in the trapezius and therefore are not well seen, although they contribute greatly to muscular detail. Their function is to retract the scapula (i.e., move the scapula together).

Front Lat Pulldown

Begin by grasping a straight bar attached to a lat pulldown machine. With your hands shoulder-width apart and palms turned forward, secure your knees under the restraint pad and fully straighten your arms so you feel a complete stretch in your lats. Maintain a slight backward tilt and keep your lower back arched throughout the move. Slowly pull the bar down to your upper chest, bringing your elbows back. Squeeze your shoulder blades together and then slowly reverse direction, returning to the start position.

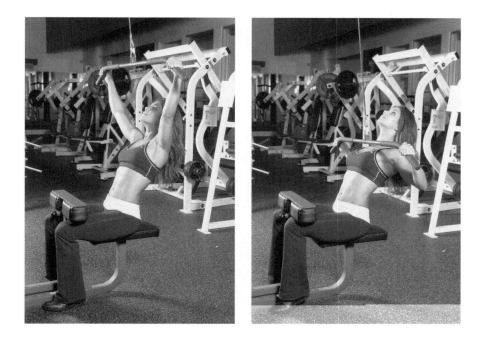

Back Exercises

One-Arm Dumbbell Row

Begin by placing your left hand and left knee on a flat bench, planting your right foot firmly on the floor. Your torso should be parallel to the ground and your lower back slightly arched. Grasp a dumbbell in your right hand with your palm facing you and let it hang by your side. Keeping your elbow close to your body, pull the dumbbell upward and back until it touches your hip. Make sure your back remains tight throughout the move. Feel a contraction in your upper back muscles and then reverse direction, slowly returning to the start position. Repeat with your left arm after finishing the desired reps.

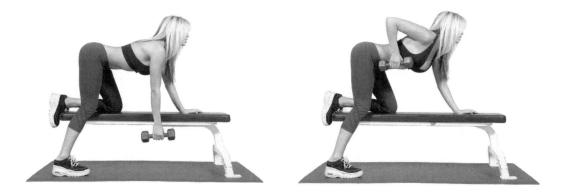

Dumbbell Pullover

Begin by lying on a flat bench. Grasp a dumbbell with both hands and raise it directly over your face. Your feet should be planted on the floor. Keeping your arms slightly bent, slowly lower the dumbbell behind your head as far as comfortably possible, feeling a complete stretch in your lats. Then, reverse direction, contracting your lats as you return to the start position.

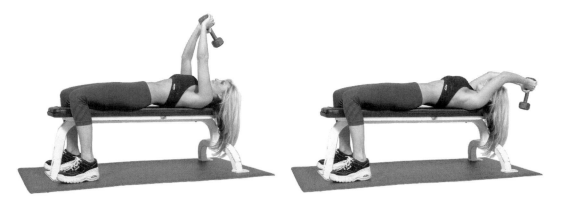

Machine Seated Row

Begin by grasping a V-bar attached to a low pulley with your palms facing each other. Place your feet against the footplate and, keeping a slight bend in your knees, sit down in front of the pulley. Fully straighten your arms so that you feel a complete stretch in your lats. Make sure your posture is erect, with a slight arch in your lower back. Slowly pull the V-bar into your lower abdomen, keeping your elbows close to your sides and your lower back tight. As the handle touches your body, squeeze your shoulder blades together and then reverse direction, slowly returning to the start position.

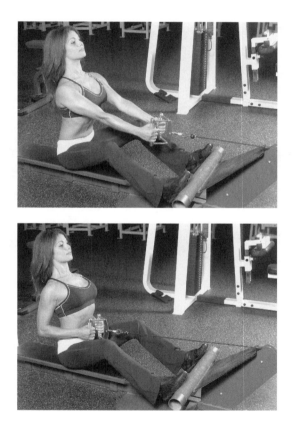

Cable Straight Arm Pulldown

Begin by taking an overhand grip on a straight bar attached to a high pulley. Slightly bend your elbows and bring the bar to eye level. Keeping a forward tilt to your upper body, slowly pull the bar down in a semicircle until it touches your upper thighs. Contract your back muscles and then reverse direction, slowly returning to the start position.

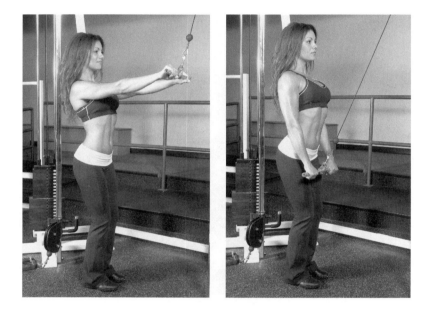

Strength Band Seated Row

Begin by grasping the loop handles of a strength band attached to a stationary object (you can use the soles of your feet, if desired), palms facing each other. Sit on the floor and maintain a slight bend to your knees. Make sure your posture is erect, with a slight arch in your lower back. Fully straighten your arms so that you feel a complete stretch in your lats (make sure there is no slack in the band). Slowly pull the handles to your lower abdomen, keeping your elbows close to your sides and your lower back slightly arched. As the handles touch your body, squeeze your shoulder blades together and then reverse direction, slowly returning to the start position.

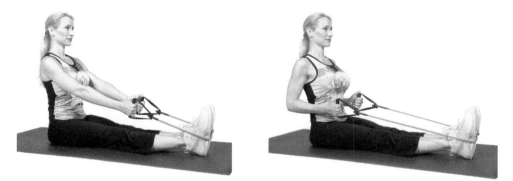

Strength Band Straight Arm Pulldown

Begin by grasping the loop handles of a strength band attached to a stationary object. Slightly bend your elbows and, with a shoulder-width grip, bring the handles to eye level. Keeping a forward tilt to your upper body, slowly pull the handles down in a semicircle until they approach your upper thighs. Contract your back muscles and then reverse direction, slowly returning to the start position.

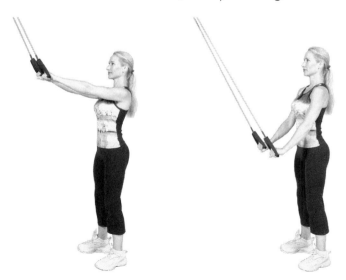

Cable Lying Pullover

Begin by lying on a flat bench placed in front of a low pulley machine. Attach a rope to the low pulley unit and grasp the rope with both hands so that your arms are at ear level. Keeping your arms slightly bent, pull the rope up in a semicircle until it is directly over your head. Contract your lats and then reverse direction, slowly returning to the start position.

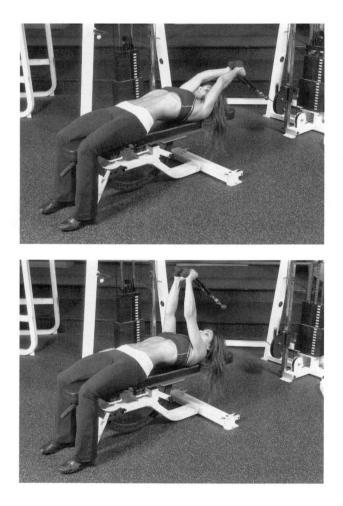

V-Bar Lat Pulldown

Begin by grasping a V-bar attached to a lat pulldown machine. Secure your knees under the restraint pad and fully straighten your arms so you feel a complete stretch in your lats. Maintain a slight backward tilt to your body and keep your lower back arched throughout the move. Slowly pull the bar to your upper chest, bringing your elbows back as you pull. Squeeze your shoulder blades together and then slowly reverse direction, returning to the start position.

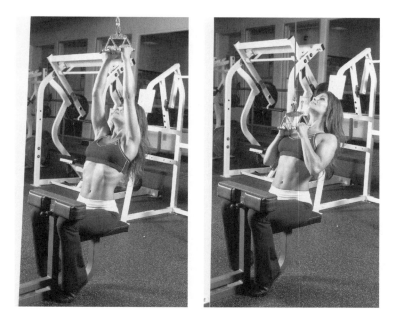

Cable Standing Reverse Low Row

Begin by grasping a straight bar attached to a low pulley. Step back from the machine and straighten your arms so you feel a stretch in your lats. Bend forward slightly at the hips for balance and keep a slight bend to your knees. Slowly pull the bar to your lower midsection, keeping your elbows close to your sides. Squeeze your shoulder blades together to contract your back muscles and then reverse direction, slowly returning to the start position.

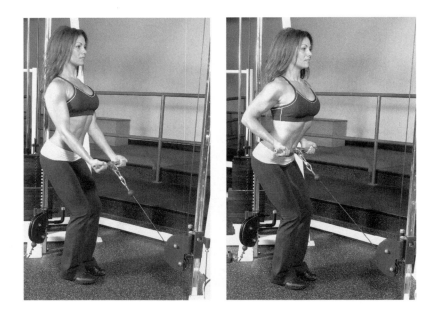

Strength Band Lying Pullover

Begin by lying on a flat bench (or the floor) and grasp the loop handles of a strength band attached to a stationary object so that your arms are at ear level. Keeping your arms slightly bent, pull the handles up in a semicircle until they are directly over your head. Contract your lats and then reverse direction, slowly returning to the start position.

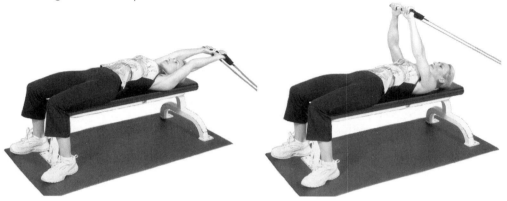

Strength Band Neutral Grip Lat Pulldown

Begin by grasping the loop handles of a strength band that is attached to a high stationary object, making sure the slack is minimal so that you achieve a complete stretch in your lats at the start position. Kneel on the floor and, with your hands close together, turn your palms so that they face each other. Maintain a slight backward tilt to your body and arch your lower back through the move. Slowly pull the handles to your upper chest, bringing your elbows back as you pull. Squeeze your shoulder blades together and then slowly reverse direction, returning to the start position.

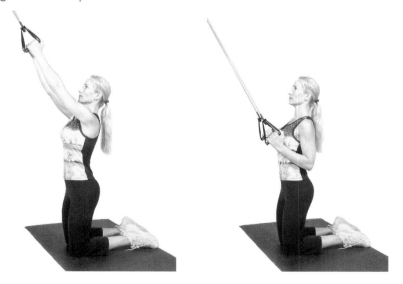

Reverse Lat Pulldown

Begin by grasping a lat pulldown bar with your hands shoulder-width apart and your palms turned toward you. Secure your knees under the restraint pad and fully straighten your arms so you feel a complete stretch in your lats. Maintain a slight backward tilt to your body and keep your lower back arched throughout the move. Slowly pull the bar to your upper chest, bringing your elbows back as you pull. Squeeze your shoulder blades together and then slowly reverse direction, returning to the start position.

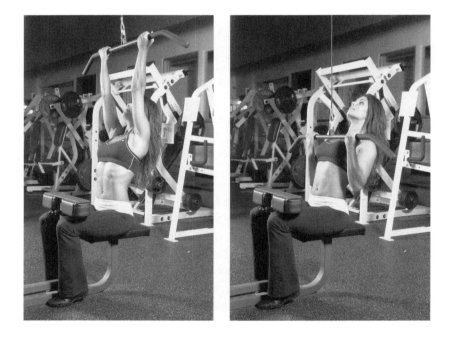

Assisted Chin-Up

Begin by standing in an assisted chin-up machine (such as a Gravitron), adjust the resistance to your abilities, and take a shoulder-width, overhand grip on the chinning bar. Fully straighten your arms so that you feel a complete stretch in your lats. Keeping your back slightly arched and your feet planted on the foot bar, slowly pull yourself up until your chin rises above the bar. Contract your lats and then slowly lower yourself to the start position.

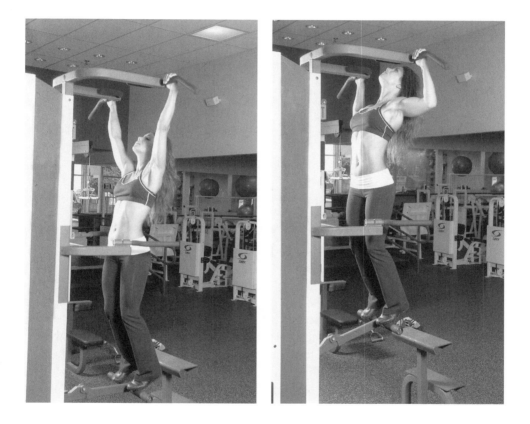

Back Exercises

Strength Band Reverse Lat Pulldown

Begin by grasping the loop handles of a strength band that is attached to a high stationary object, making sure the slack is minimal so that you achieve a complete stretch in your lats at the start position. Kneel on the floor and, with your hands shoulder-width apart, turn your palms so that they face your body. Maintain a slight backward tilt to your body and arch your lower back through the move. Slowly pull the handles to your upper chest, bringing your elbows back as you pull. Squeeze your shoulder blades together and then slowly reverse direction, returning to the start position.

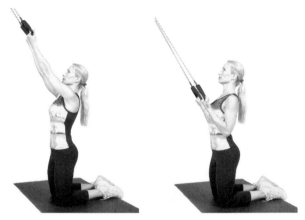

Strength Band Overhand Lat Pulldown

Begin by grasping the loop handles of a strength band that is attached to a high stationary object, making sure the slack is minimal so that you achieve a complete stretch in your lats at the start position. Kneel on the floor and, with your hands shoulder-width apart, turn your palms so that they face away from your body. Maintain a slight backward tilt to your body and arch your lower back through the move. Slowly pull the handles to your upper chest, bringing your elbows back as you pull. Squeeze your shoulder blades together and then slowly reverse direction, returning to the start position.

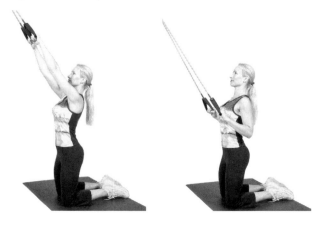

Cross Cable Pulldown

Begin by grasping the loop handles of a high pulley apparatus. Kneel on the floor facing away from the apparatus and allow your arms to extend fully so that you feel a stretch in your lat muscles. Your palms should face away from your body and your lower back should be slightly arched. Keeping your body stable, pull the handles down and toward your sides, turning your palms in on the descent. Contract your lats and then slowly reverse direction, returning to the start position.

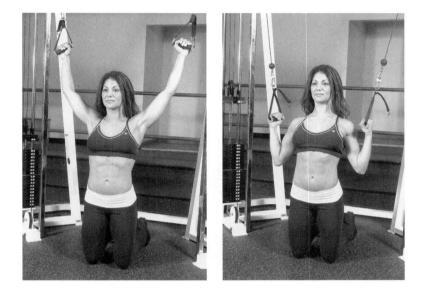

Back Exercises

One-Arm Cable Standing Low Row

Begin by grasping the loop handle of a low pulley with your right hand, using a neutral grip (palm facing in). Step back from the machine and straighten your right arm so you feel a stretch in your right lat. Keep your right leg back and bend your left leg so your weight is forward. Place your left hand on your left knee for balance (or, if desired, hold on to the machine with your left hand). Slowly pull the loop handle toward your right side, keeping your elbow close. Contract your right lat and then reverse direction, slowly returning to the starting position. Repeat with your left arm after finishing the desired reps on your right.

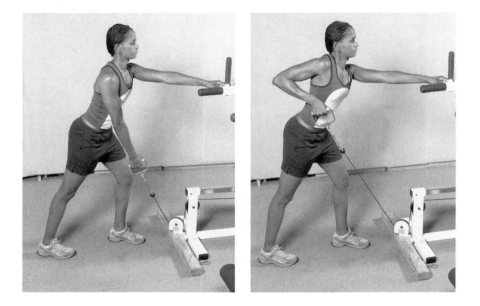

Strength Band High Lat Pull

Begin by grasping the loop handles of a strength band attached to a high stationary object, using a reverse grip (palms facing up). Take a shoulder-width stance, step back, and straighten your arms so you feel a stretch in your lats. Keep your body erect and motionless throughout the move. Slowly pull the handles toward your body so that your elbows travel back as far as possible, keeping your elbows close to your sides at all times. Contract your back muscles and then slowly return the handles along the same path back to the start position.

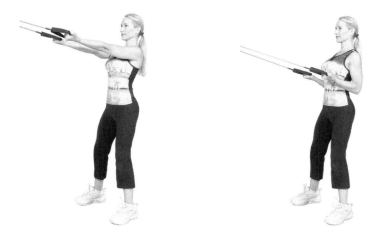

One-Arm Strength Band Standing Low Row

Begin by grasping the loop handle of a strength band attached to a low stationary object, using a neutral grip (palm facing in). Step back and straighten your right arm so you feel a stretch in your right lat. Keep your right leg back and bend your left leg so your weight is forward. For balance, place your left hand on your left knee or hold on to a stationary object. Slowly pull the loop handle toward your right side, keeping your elbow close. Contract your right lat and then reverse direction, slowly returning to the starting position. Repeat with your left arm after finishing the desired reps on your right.

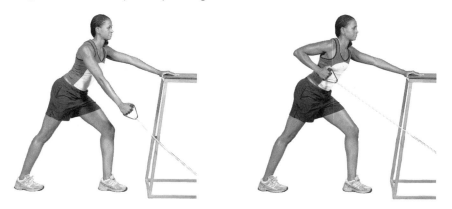

Abdominals

The abdominal complex is made up of four distinct muscles: the rectus abdominis, external obliques, internal obliques, and transverse abdominis. Let's take a look at their form and function.

The rectus abdominis is one long sheath of muscle that runs from just underneath the breastbone (sternum) all the way down into the pelvis. There is a prevailing misconception that the upper and lower portions of the rectus abdominis are two separate muscles that can be trained independently of one another; this is not the case. Because of its configuration, the entire complex contracts as a single unit. Consequently, you cannot work one part without affecting the rest of the muscle. However, by altering the point where spinal movement occurs, it is possible to accentuate one aspect more than another.

The obliques consist of two separate muscles: the external obliques and the internal obliques. These are the "waist" muscles that run diagonally along the sides of your body. When properly developed, they give your waist a sleek, firm appearance. The external obliques are the more visible of the two muscles, spanning from the upper part of your ribs all the way down to your hips. The internal obliques lie underneath the external obliques and thus are somewhat hidden from view. For the most part, both muscles work together as a unit, helping to bend or twist your torso sideways.

The transversus abdominis lies deep within your abdomen. Although it is not outwardly visible on the body, the transversus abdominis plays a central role in containing your internal organs as well as assisting in pulmonary function. Because of its position, direct stress really cannot be applied to this muscle. It does, however, act as a stabilizer in the performance of many abdominal exercises and thus receives considerable ancillary stress during training.

Twisting Crunch

Begin by lying face up on the floor with your knees bent. Your thighs should be perpendicular to the ground and your hands should be folded across your chest. Slowly raise your shoulders up and forward toward your chest, twisting your body to the right. Feel a contraction in your abdominal muscles and then slowly reverse direction, returning to the start position. After performing the desired number of repetitions, repeat the process, twisting your body to the left. Or, if you prefer, you can alternate from one side to the other until the desired number of reps are completed.

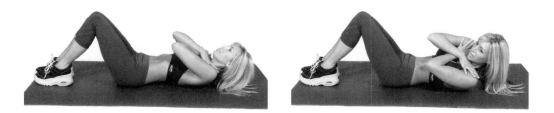

Leg Lowering

Begin by lying on the floor with your hands at your sides and feet together. Extend your legs as high as possible and bring your lower body off the floor, starting with your lower back and proceeding to your mid-back. Breathe in at the top of the move and slowly roll back down in sequential fashion, exhaling as you descend.

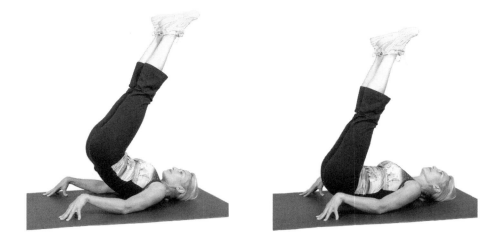

Hanging Knee Raise

Begin by grasping a chinning bar with a shoulder-width grip or by placing your arms in abdominal straps. Keeping your knees bent, slowly raise your legs upward, lifting your butt so that your pelvis tilts toward your stomach. Contract your abs and then reverse direction, returning your legs to the start position. Keep your upper torso motionless throughout the exercise. For increased intensity, straighten your legs while performing the move.

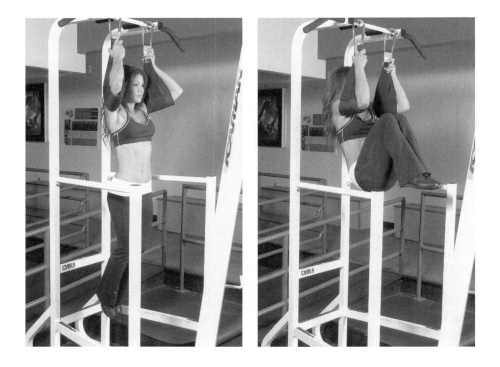

Cable Kneeling Rope Crunch

Begin by kneeling in front of a high pulley apparatus with your body facing the machine. Grasp the ends of a rope attached to the pulley and keep your elbows in toward your ears. Keeping your lower back immobile, slowly curl your body downward, bringing your elbows down toward your knees. Contract your abs and then slowly uncurl your body, returning to the start position.

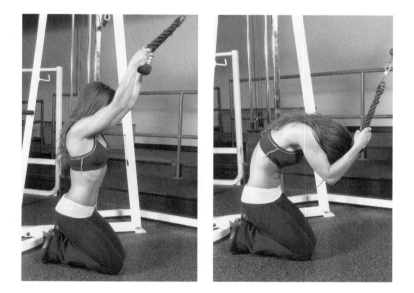

Abdominal Exercises

Strength Band Kneeling Crunch

Begin by grasping the loop handles of a strength band attached to a stationary object. Kneel down and keep your elbows pressed in at your ears. Keeping your lower back straight, slowly curl your upper torso downward as far as comfortably possible, bringing your elbows toward your knees. Contract your abs and then slowly uncurl your body, returning to the start position.

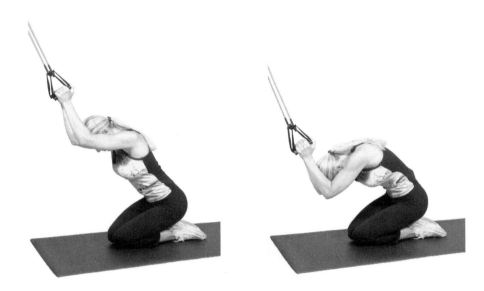

Crunch

Begin by lying face up on the floor with your feet planted firmly on the floor. Keep your knees bent and your hands folded across your chest. Keeping your lower back pressed to the floor, slowly raise your shoulders up and forward toward your chest, shortening the distance of your trunk. Feel a contraction in your abdominal muscles and then slowly reverse direction, returning to the start position.

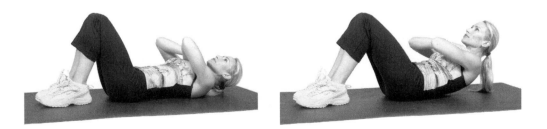

Reverse Curl

Begin by lying on the floor with hands at your sides. Curl your knees into your stomach and lift your butt so that it is slightly off the ground. Keeping your upper back pressed into the floor at all times, raise your butt as high as possible so that your pelvis tilts toward your chest. Contract your abs and then reverse direction, returning to the start position.

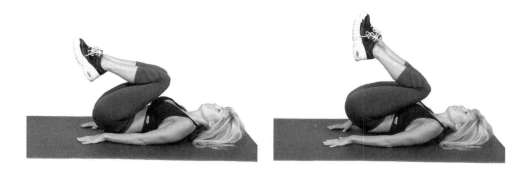

Side Jackknife

Lie on your left side with your feet together. Make a fist with your right hand and keep it pressed to your right ear. Simultaneously raise your right leg and torso toward each other as far as comfortably possible. Contract your oblique muscles and then slowly reverse direction and return to the start position. After performing the prescribed number of repetitions, repeat the process on the left.

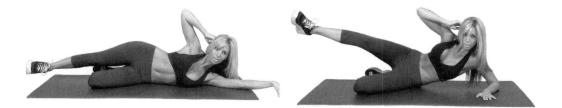

Abdominal Exercises

Toe Touch

Begin by lying flat on the floor with your arms and legs straight in the air, perpendicular to your body. Slowly curl your torso up and forward, raising your hands as close to your toes as possible. Contract your abs and then reverse direction, returning to the start position.

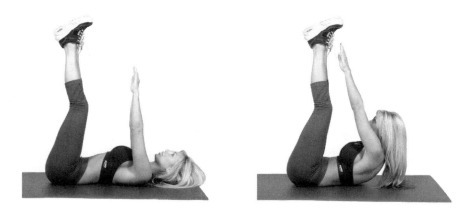

Pedaling

Begin by lying on the floor with your legs bent at a 90-degree angle. Ball your hands into fists and place them at your ears (not behind your head!). Slowly bring your right knee up toward your left elbow and try to touch them to one another. As you return your right leg and left elbow to the start position, bring your left leg toward your right elbow in the same manner. Continue this movement, alternating between right and left sides as if pedaling a bike.

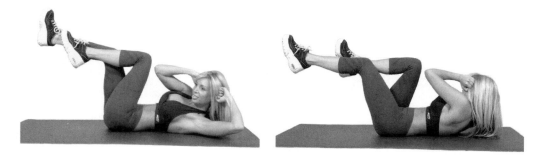

Supplements

11

No topic on fitness draws more interest than that of supplementation. After all, who wouldn't like to take a "magic pill" that can increase energy, burn fat, and build lean muscle? Certainly I would! In truth, however, there is no easy way to a great body. Upward of 95 percent of your results will be achieved through proper training, nutrition, and rest. Provided you eat right, train hard, and allow for adequate recuperation—as outlined in my shapeover program—you'll develop a terrific physique over time.

That said, to eke out that last 5 percent of your genetic potential, supplements can be beneficial. When properly utilized, they provide an extra boost that helps you attain your personal best.

Unfortunately, most supplements are of limited value; many are little more than snake oil. Yet that hasn't stopped unscrupulous hucksters from making outrageous, unfounded claims about their products. You see, for all intents and purposes, the supplement industry is largely unregulated. Provided a product does not claim to treat or cure disease, its manufacturer can pretty much say whatever it wants without fear of reprisal. It's the ultimate case of buyer beware.

So how do you go about deciding which supplements to take and which to avoid? The decision should come down to a cost–benefit analysis; namely, do the benefits outweigh the costs. And cost is not just a function of money. Although supplements can be a drain on your wallet, the potential adverse effects on health can be of an even greater concern. Remember, just because a supplement claims to be "herbal" or "all natural" doesn't mean it's safe. Cyanide, arsenic, and hemlock are natural substances that can be lethal, even in small doses. Moreover, certain supplements can have negative interactions with various medications you might use. These factors need to be balanced against the efficacy of the product.

With this in mind, let's discuss some supplements that may be of value in your quest to shape over your body. I will cover only supplements that are supported by peer-reviewed research as well as proven to be of benefit in my own experience working with clients from all walks of life. Make sure to evaluate the products vis-à-vis your own individual needs and consult with your physician when appropriate.

Vitamins and Minerals

Vitamins and minerals are the most popular supplements on the market. Nearly one-half of all revenues of the supplement industry are attributable to sales of these micronutrients. But is their supplementation really necessary? The simple answer is: it depends.

If you eat a balanced diet *and* eat a sufficient quantity of food, then it's likely you are getting the recommended daily allowance (RDA) of all the necessary vitamins and minerals. (Although there is still the possibility that you can be missing out on a particular one, depending on the specific composition of your meals.) Assuming you aren't deficient in micronutrient intake, then there is no additional benefit in taking a multivitamin because your body can't store the excess for future use.

On the other hand, if you tend to eat a lot of the same foods, or if you are dieting and your calorie intake falls below maintenance level, then there's a good chance that you are nutrient deficient. Vitamins and minerals are essential to your health and well-being as well as to your exercise performance and ability to burn fat. They facilitate energy transfer, prevent disease, and act as coenzymes to assist in many chemical reactions. A significant deficiency in any of these micronutrients can lead to severe illness. For instance, a lack of niacin results in pellagra.

My personal recommendation is to take a daily multivitamin and mineral complex regardless of your dietary habits. Short of having regular blood tests, it's very difficult to know whether you are lacking in any of the micronutrients (calcium and folate can be especially difficult to acquire through normal dietary means), and a good multivitamin acts as an insurance policy against any possible deficiencies. And there's really no downside: the cost is minimal and any micronutrients not utilized by your body are simply excreted in your urine without ill effect.

In addition to taking a multivitamin, there is a class of micronutrients called antioxidants that require additional supplementation, over and above the U.S. government's recommended daily allowance. Understand that the RDA was established to prevent deficiencies, not to improve overall health and wellness, and antioxidants have benefits beyond their basic functions.

What's so special about antioxidants? Well, they are the body's scavengers, helping to defend against damage caused by free radicals—unstable molecules that can injure healthy cells and tissues. Every time you breathe, oxygen uptake causes free radical production. Environmental factors such as pollutants, smoke, and certain chemicals also contribute to their formation. If left unchecked, they can wreak havoc on your physique and cause a multitude of ailments including arthritis, cardiovascular disease, dementia, and cancer.

Here's a short course in how the process works: Your body is made up of billions of cells held together by a series of electronic bonds. These bonds are arranged in pairs so that one electron balances the other. However, in response to various occurrences (such as oxygen consumption), a molecule can lose one of its electron pairs, making it an unstable free radical. The free radical then tries to replace its lost electron by stealing one from another molecule. This sets up a chain reaction where the second molecule becomes a free radical and attacks a third molecule, which becomes a free radical and attacks a fourth molecule, and so on.

To prevent rampant free radical production, your body has a sophisticated internal antioxidant system. Various antioxidant enzymes combine with antioxidants from the foods you eat to help keep free radicals at bay. But when free radical activity reaches a critical level, the system can become overwhelmed, causing damage to cellular tissues.

Physical activity only exacerbates the situation. Because of increased oxygen consumption, free radical production skyrockets during exercise (by as much as twenty-fold over resting levels), overwhelming the body's internal defense system. If left unchecked, this results in an inflammation of muscle tissue, impairing muscular function and slowing recovery. Thus, active people have an even greater need for antioxidant supplementation.

Although there are dozens of known antioxidants, two are absolutely indispensable: vitamins C and E. These vitamins are partners in defense; they have a synergistic relationship, working together so that their combined effect is greater than the sum of their individual actions. Other antioxidants such as alpha-lipoic acid, coenzyme Q10, selenium, and carotenoids are also beneficial; they not only have important health benefits in their own right, but can actually help to regenerate the activity of vitamins C and E as well.

Although antioxidants can be obtained through dietary means, it's virtually impossible to consume adequate quantities from food sources alone. For example, you'd have to drink 11 glasses of orange juice to get your daily vitamin C requirement or chow down over three pounds of almonds for the necessary amount of vitamin E! And because it has been shown that at low doses (even above RDA guidelines) antioxidants don't provide adequate protection against infirmity, supplementation isn't an option—it's a necessity. Given that side effects are virtually nonexistent at suggested levels, there is very little risk and great potential reward.

Table 11.1   Recommended Dosages for Antioxidants

Antioxidant	Dosage
Vitamin C	800 mg
Vitamin E	400 IU
Coenzyme Q10	50 mg
Alpha-lipoic acid	100 mg
Polyphenols	50 mg
Lycopene	10 mg
Selenium	200 mcg

As a rule, it is best to consume supplemental vitamins and minerals in conjunction with a meal. The absorption of micronutrients is improved when they are taken with food. This also improves gastrointestinal tolerance of the supplement.

Table 11.1 lists some of the most important antioxidants and their prescribed dosages. Although you can buy each of these antioxidants separately, it is generally more cost effective and convenient to buy a single supplement that has all of these ingredients. Look for a respected brand to ensure good quality.

Fat Burners

Weight-loss aids account for about one-third of all supplement sales. Often called "fat burners" or "thermogenics," these products purport to strip away fat safely and easily. Unfortunately, most of these products have little or no efficacy. At best, they act as mild appetite suppressants; at worst, they can cause grave side effects.

The most controversial fat-burner supplements are those that contain ephedra, an herb extracted from the ma huang plant, as their active ingredient. Ephedra has a long track record in Chinese medicine, with its use dating back more than 5,000 years. Today, ephedra alkaloids—derivatives that have a similar chemical structure to ephedra—are found in a wide array of over-the-counter medications, including those that treat allergies, colds, and asthma.

Ephedra functions much like an amphetamine (and is actually the raw material used to manufacture methamphetamine), having a dual action on fat loss. First, it stimulates the central nervous system to promote the release of catecholamines (adrenaline and noradrenaline). These catecholamines then bind to your beta receptors—the "exit doors" that allow fat to be released from adipocytes—stimulating the breakdown of fat. Second, it functions as a "beta agonist," making your beta receptors more receptive to the catecholamines. In combination, this shifts your body into a fat-burning mode, heightening thermogenesis.

Ephedrine also is a powerful appetite suppressant. By stimulating the ventromedial hypothalamus—the area of the brain linked to satiety—it causes a neurochemical cascade that ultimately reduces food cravings. Researchers estimate that 75 percent of ephedrine-induced weight loss is due to these anorectic effects.

But although ephedra has been proven to be efficacious, it can cause adverse side effects. As with amphetamines, it has a stimulant effect, producing a buzz that can last for hours. It is common to experience palpitations, insomnia, dry mouth, headaches, dizziness, tremors, and sexual dysfunction when first taking the supplement. In some people these symptoms go away after several weeks; in others, they don't.

Other complications from ephedra can be more serious, even lethal. In rare cases, strokes, seizures, and heart attacks have been reported. And because of its tendency to raise blood pressure and heart rate, ephedra is explicitly contraindicated for anyone with hypertension or existing cardiac anomalies.

Given the potential downside, you should always consult with a physician before taking an ephedra-based product. He or she can evaluate your situation, making sure there are no contraindications and that it doesn't interfere with any medication you might be taking. Also be aware that ephedra has come under legal scrutiny and may be banned in your state.

A safer supplemental alternative for fat loss is green tea extract. Green tea extract has two modes of action. First, it contains caffeine, which exerts its effects by acting on the sympathetic nervous system to increase catecholamine (i.e., epinephrine and norepinephrine) production. As previously noted, catecholamines facilitate the release of free fatty acids from adipocytes, allowing fat to be utilized for short-term energy.

Second, it contains compounds called catechins that serve to further increase metabolism. Catechins inhibit an enzyme (called catechol-O-methyl-transferase) that is responsible for degrading noradrenaline, a potent hormone that promotes the oxidation of body fat. In combination, caffeine and catechins act synergistically to enhance resting energy expenditure beyond what is achieved by caffeine alone.

As an added benefit, green tea enhances your well being. It is replete in vitamins, minerals, and antioxidants and, because of its concentration of flavonoids, can even help to increase bone density and stave off cardiovascular disease!

Understand, though, the effects of green tea on fat burning are relatively modest. Don't expect significant weight loss. At best, it gives a slight boost to your slimming efforts, helping to shed a few extra pounds.

You can take green tea either in pill form or by brewing herbal green tea leaves into a beverage. If you choose to consume it as a drink, refrain from adding cream or sugar. Doing so offsets the increase in metabolic rate and the fat-burning benefits are lost. If plain tea is simply too bitter for your taste buds, then try using skim milk or artificial sweeteners as flavor enhancers.

Also, it's generally best to abstain from using any caffeinated product in the hours before bedtime. Because of its stimulatory effects, it can interfere with your circadian rhythms and throw your sleep–wake cycle out of whack. This leads to desynchronization of your biorhythms, a condition where sleep is less restful at night and mental acuity is compromised during the day.

On a final note, understand that fat burners only work in conjunction with caloric restriction; you must adhere to a proper diet and exercise program to achieve effects. Despite the hype, you can't just take a pill or potion, sit back, and watch the fat melt away.

Using Caffeine Safely

Caffeine is often cited as a health hazard. It has been linked to everything from heart disease to cancer and is even lumped together with alcohol and nicotine as the "dangerous triad." Many health spas refrain from serving caffeinated products because of its reputed ill effects.

The truth, however, is that caffeine has gotten a bad rap. A close examination of peer-reviewed research reveals that any carcinogenic effects of caffeine have been vastly overstated. Studies showing a positive correlation between caffeine and cancer were plagued by errors in statistical analysis and flawed research design (one of the most cited studies gave lab rats enormous quantities of caffeine—far beyond what the average person could ever consume). When all the available information is examined, there's really no evidence that modest caffeine consumption causes any detriments to overall well being. In fact, several studies have actually found that caffeine may have a negative effect on certain forms of cancer!

Now I'm certainly not advocating that you load up on caffeinated beverages. Caffeine is a stimulant. At high doses, it can cause a host of unwanted side effects such as hypertension, nervousness, insomnia, and gastrointestinal distress. Guzzling mass quantities of coffee and soda will only make you wired and irritable—not lean and defined.

However, when used in moderation, caffeine can be a safe and effective way to expedite a loss of body fat. In the form of green tea, it is certainly something to consider if you are seeking an extra boost in fat-burning capacity.

Omega-3 Fat

In the not-too-distant past, nutritionists counseled against consuming dietary fat. The battle cry of "eat fat and you'll get fat" resonated with the U.S. public and an entire industry arose to produce a myriad of no-fat products that dominated supermarket shelves.

Now, after years of watching the obesity epidemic spiral out of control, we know this advice was misguided. Ultra-low-fat diets are not only unnecessary, but they are also counterproductive to achieving optimal health and body composition. Fat is an essential nutrient and plays a vital role in many bodily functions. It is involved in cushioning your internal organs for protection; aiding in the absorption of vitamins; and facilitating the production of cell membranes, hormones, and prostaglandins. Physiologically, it would be impossible to survive without the inclusion of fat in your diet.

The most important dietary fats are those that are polyunsaturated. Because we lack certain enzymes, polyunsaturated fats (PUFAs) cannot be manufactured by the human body, so they are an essential component in food. A deficiency ultimately causes a breakdown in cellular function, leading to a host of anomalies including bloody urine, fatty liver, and even reproductive disorders.

Of the types of polyunsaturated fat (PUFA), the most important is the *omega-3* fat. Omega-3 has been proven to confer numerous health-related benefits. For one, it exerts a substantial cardioprotective effect, inhibiting the production of LDL (the "bad" cholesterol) and increasing the production of HDL (the "good" cholesterol). Research has shown that this translates into a significant decrease in cardiovascular mortality, reducing death from coronary events by as much as 70 percent. There is also evidence that omega-3 might play a role in suppressing various cancers, inflammatory diseases, and a host of other ailments. It's as close to a nutritional panacea as there is.

What's more, omega-3 plays a role in reducing body fat. Because it is so biologically active, the body prefers to use it to fuel cellular functions and won't store it as fat until these functions are satisfied. Moreover, it acts as a fuel partitioner, directing fatty acids away from storage and toward oxidation. One of the ways this is accomplished is through enzyme regulation. Specifically, omega-3 helps to increase the activity of fat-burning enzymes and suppress the activity of fat-storing enzymes. The net effect is better fat metabolism and improved body composition.

Additionally, omega-3 increases the levels of a class of fat-burning compounds called uncoupling proteins (UCPs). UCPs act on various bodily tissues to heighten thermogenesis, allowing calories to be burned off immediately as heat rather than stored as fat. Unfortunately, these substances are often suppressed, especially in those who are overweight. By revving up UCP activity, PUFA shifts your body into a fat-burning mode, promoting a leaner physique.

I have designed the shapeover meal plans to be rich in omega-3 fat. There is a daily dose of flaxseed oil (one of the richest sources of omega-3) and several weekly servings of cold-water fish (the most abundant source of omega-3 derivatives). However, for those who do not like to eat fish or cannot stomach flaxseed oil, supplementation with fish oil capsules is recommended. The capsules provide an easy method of consumption and, as opposed to the fish from which they are derived, tend to be mercury free, thus making for a potentially safer alternative. A 5- to 10-gram dose is recommended, using a formula of 1 gram for every 20 pounds of body weight (each capsule is usually 1 gram). It is generally best to split consumption into two doses, taking half in the morning and the other half at night.

Fiber

Fiber is perhaps the most unheralded of all nutrients. There is a large body of scientific evidence indicating that a diet high in fiber is beneficial to your well being. Among its numerous health-related benefits are that it helps to maintain bowel regularity, stave off the growth of malignant tumors, reduce serum cholesterol levels, and improve the ratio of "good" to "bad" cholesterol.

Best of all, fiber is unique in that it cannot be completely digested (because the body lacks an enzyme called cellulose that's responsible for breaking down fiber in the gastrointestinal system) and therefore passes directly into the colon unimpeded. Hence, you can eat more without having it stored in your system. In fact, it has been reported that by simply doubling fiber intake from 18 to 36 grams, you reduce the available calories in your diet by more than 100 calories per day! Bottom line: fiber can't make you gain weight!

Fiber is found in a wide array of carb-based foods, especially unrefined grains, fruits, and vegetables. Fiber intake should exceed 20 grams per 1,000 calories consumed, with a minimum of 30 grams per day. Although I've included healthy amounts of fibrous foods in the shapeover meal plans, there is a possibility (depending on caloric intake and food substitutions) that you still might not get the suggested daily intake. If this is the case, I recommend that you take a fiber supplement. They are quick and convenient, allowing you to boost your fiber intake without a great deal of hassle. The supplements come in a variety of modes, including the traditional powdered form (which is mixed with water or soft food), as well as wafers, tablets, and capsules. If you have a sensitive stomach, check with your physician to see which one is right for you.

Muscle Builders

Over the years, people have consumed everything from deer antler to rhinoceros testicles in an effort to put on a little extra muscle. Suffice to say, none of these products worked very well! Then along came creatine, and muscle-building supplements were revolutionized almost overnight.

Creatine is a nutrient synthesized from three amino acids: arginine, glycine, and methionine. Approximately 95 percent of your creatine supply is stored in muscle tissue, with the rest located primarily in your heart and brain. Its primary function is to work in conjunction with the high-energy compound ATP, fueling muscular contractions during intense exercise.

The problem, however, is that your body has limited stores of creatine and, once its supply is exhausted, muscles begin to fatigue. This is where supplementation has proven to be effective. By allowing larger stores of creatine to build up in muscle tissue, you are able to exercise longer and harder. This is especially beneficial during weight training. With more creatine available, you can squeeze out a few extra reps per set. And this increased training capacity translates into an ability to build more muscle.

Creatine also helps to build muscle by promoting cellular hydration. You see, when creatine is stored in muscles, it pulls in water along with it. This causes the muscles to swell, which stimulates protein synthesis and inhibits protein breakdown—the basis for muscular development. Better yet, since creatine is primarily stored in fast-twitch fibers—the ones with the greatest potential for growth—its muscle-building effects are heightened.

Before you run out and stock up on the product, however, understand that creatine isn't going to miraculously transform your physique. Most users can expect to add no more than a few pounds of lean muscle tissue, even under ideal conditions. Furthermore, creatine doesn't work for everybody. About 30 percent of the population are "nonresponders" who achieve little or no benefit from creatine supplementation. This seems to be dependent on your body's internal creatine stores and the type of diet you consume. Because beef is high in creatine content, those people who eat red meat will tend to have higher creatine stores and thus be less responsive; vegetarians, on the other hand, will tend to see better results.

On the plus side, creatine is virtually free from side effects. Other than a few isolated reports of muscle cramping, no other symptoms have been associated with its use. It can, however, be associated with subcutaneous water retention, so this must be factored into the equation and balanced with your desire to maximize muscle gain.

Creatine is traditionally taken in two phases: a loading phase (to thoroughly saturate the muscles with creatine) followed by a maintenance phase (to keep creatine stores full). That said, I've found that taking a daily dose of 5 grams for one month serves the same purpose as loading without the hassle of frequent consumption.

Ideally, creatine should be consumed with a high-glycemic carbohydrate drink such as grape or cranberry juice. The associated insulin response helps to drive creatine into your muscles, maximizing its storage. Taking it along with your postexercise meal is generally the best way to go because this way you can get double-duty out of the "window of opportunity."

Although creatine comes in several different forms, stick with pure creatine monohydrate. There is no evidence that alternatives such as effervescent or liquid creatine have any additional benefits and they are much more expensive. And don't think that increasing intake over and above these levels will increase the benefits; once your stores are saturated, the body cannot stockpile additional creatine for future use and any excess is simply excreted from the body through the urine.

12

Beyond the 28-Day Program

Congratulations! You've finished the four-week program and should now be significantly more firm and toned than when you started. Your body fat should be down, your energy levels up, and you should feel good about your progress. Best of all, you've done it in a safe and healthy manner that will have nothing but positive effects on your well-being.

My 28-Day Shapeover regimen, however, isn't just a short-term solution to your fitness goals; it can be used over and over again for continued results. The periodized nature of the program makes it ideal for avoiding training plateaus, allowing you to shape your body to its fullest potential. Still, like any routine, it will need to be tweaked based on your individual goals, abilities, and progress. Here are some things to keep in mind when going forward.

Changing the Split

In accordance with the principle of maintaining fitness variety, you should vary the split of your routine every few months or so. The more you change your training variables, the more you keep your body off guard, forcing it to adapt by getting stronger and harder.

There are many ways to split your routine and virtually any combination of muscle groups can be employed depending on your preference. For example:

- You can do a push–pull split where you train chest, shoulders, and triceps on Day 1 (the pushing muscles); quadriceps, hamstrings, and calves on

Day 2 (lower body); and then back, biceps, and abs on Day 3 (the pulling muscles).

- You can do a front, back, and side split where you train chest, quadriceps, and abs on Day 1 (front of body); back, hamstrings, and calves on Day 2 (back of body); and shoulders, biceps, and triceps on Day 3 (side of body).
- You can do a rotating split, where different combinations are alternated from week to week.

Again, you have a myriad of groupings to choose from. Experiment with different splits and see which ones work best for you. Remember, variety is the spice of fitness—mix it up as much as possible!

Prioritizing Your Routine

As a general rule, it is best to train larger muscle groups before smaller ones. Because small muscles tend to fatigue more easily, training them first can compromise your ability to work their larger counterparts. This is particularly true when the smaller muscle acts as a secondary mover in a compound movement (i.e., the biceps in the lat pulldown, the triceps in the incline chest press, etc.).

That said, rules are often made to be broken and this one is no exception. Once you have achieved a sufficient degree of muscular development, it is beneficial to prioritize your routine so that lagging muscles are trained first in your workouts, regardless of their size. Understand that lifting weights is an extremely demanding activity. As you go through a workout, your energy levels gradually will be sapped of strength, leaving you physically and mentally depleted. It is therefore only natural that you won't be able to generate the same intensity on the last few exercises you perform as you will in the beginning of your session. By prioritizing lagging muscles, you'll ensure that they are worked to their fullest potential and thereby maximize their development.

For example, if your hamstrings are a problem area, train them before quadriceps; if your abs need work, train them before back and chest. In this way, you'll get the best workout for the muscles that need it the most, improving your shape and symmetry.

The task of determining lagging muscle groups is an ongoing process. You should constantly evaluate your physique with an eye toward creating total symmetry, where each muscle flows into the next like a sculpture. This is not only important from an aesthetic standpoint, but from a functional standpoint as well. Structural imbalances reduce muscular efficiency, making you more prone to injuries to the muscles and connective tissue. If nothing else, a training injury can prevent you from working out, perhaps for a lengthy period of time. And remember, if you can't train, you can't shape your body to its fullest potential!

Targeting a Rep Range

You can utilize a variety of repetition ranges to attain various fitness goals. Although there are certain physical and genetic limitations as to what you ultimately can achieve, the following general rules apply in respect to repetition ranges:

- A set of up to 4 repetitions (using weights in excess of 90 percent of your 1-repetition maximum) is best for increasing brute strength. This is considered a low repetition range and is oriented to powerlifting goals.

- A set of 8 to 12 repetitions (using weights of about 70 percent of your 1-repetition maximum) is best for increasing overall muscularity. This is considered a moderate repetition range and is oriented toward developing a bodybuilding physique.

- A set of 15 to 20 repetitions (using weights of about 50 percent of your 1-repetition maximum) is best for increasing local muscular endurance. This rep range is oriented toward achieving lean muscle tone without significantly increasing muscular bulk.

With this in mind, you should adapt your use of repetitions according to your needs. Understand that you don't have to choose a rep range and then employ it for all muscle groups. Rather, you can and should be selective, using repetitions specific to your concept of how you want your body to look. Think of your body as a sculpture and you as the body sculptor. Within your genetic potential, you have the power to shape your body just about any way you choose.

For example, let's say you're happy with your biceps development but not with that of your triceps. The solution: utilize a moderate rep scheme (i.e., 8 to 12 reps) for your triceps while keeping reps high for your biceps training. Over time, this should help to develop your triceps to the point that they "catch up" with your biceps. The same approach should be applied to all your muscle groups, taking into account how they mesh with one another. If your quadriceps tend to overpower your hamstrings, go with high reps for the quads and moderate reps for the hams; if your back eclipses your chest, use high reps for the back and moderate reps for the chest. By employing the proper repetition range for your goals, you'll go a long way toward sculpting your physique just the way you want it to appear.

Taking a Break

Because of the intense nature of this routine, it will be necessary to monitor your body for signs of overtraining on an ongoing basis. Overtraining is a complicated subject that involves both psychological and physiological factors (see "Understanding Overtraining" on page 55 for an overview of its symptoms), and you need to be continually in tune with your body and listen to its needs. The demands of high-energy training combined with external factors (such as sleeping patterns, stress levels, nutritional deficiencies, and other circumstances) can sometimes be overwhelming, necessitating an extra day or two of rest. Therefore, if you feel weak or run-down and need an extra day off, take it! If you can't train at a sufficient level of intensity, it is better to rest a day and come back stronger the next.

You mustn't allow the psychological drive to achieve your fitness goals to interfere with better judgment. Although there is a natural temptation to feel you can't miss a workout at any cost, this line of thinking most often is counterproductive. Don't lose sight of the fact that recuperation is what ultimately produces physical gains, not the act of training itself. For optimal results, be dispassionate in your approach and train scientifically, not haphazardly.

To help ensure that you give your body time for sufficient recovery, it is advisable to take a full week off from training every three months or so. This will allow your body to "heal" itself, reducing the incidence of injury from overuse and helping to stave off the possibility of reaching a training plateau. Invariably, you'll come back better and stronger after this respite, able to train at peak intensity.

Should you become overtrained, you'll need to stop training for a minimum of about two weeks, and perhaps more, depending on severity. Complete rest from exercise is the only cure for overtraining; even light cardiovascular exercise is taboo. Err on the side of caution here: should you come back too soon, you'll only set back your progress indefinitely.

Supplementation with antioxidants is particularly important when you are overtrained. Overtraining causes rampant free radical production, exacerbating the catabolic effects on your body. As discussed in chapter 11, this can lead to a host of undesirable effects on bodily processes, some of them potentially serious. Make antioxidant supplementation part of your daily routine and you'll go a long way toward reducing the consequences of overtraining, keeping yourself healthy and fit over the long haul.

Supplementation with glutamine also can be of some value during periods of overtraining. Glutamine is the most abundant free amino acid in human muscle and plasma, and is utilized at high rates by immune cells (especially leukocytes). During periods of catabolic stress such as overtraining, glutamine levels fall precipitously and remain suppressed for the duration of the condition. This reduces the immune response, making you particularly vulnerable to illnesses such as respiratory infection, fever, and other types of sickness. Although glutamine is synthesized internally by your body, its production might not be enough to support immune function when bodily stress is high. Therefore, if you are overtrained, consider taking a daily dose of glutamine—about .2 grams per pound of body weight. For a 120-pound woman, this would equate to approximately 24 grams per day.

Refeeding Your Body

To maintain consistently low levels of body fat, you should include a regularly scheduled "refeed" day in your dietary regimen. Think of the refeed as a cheat day, where you can eat pretty much anything you want, including sugar or fat-laden foods. Within reason, there are no dietary restrictions. Go ahead and order a pizza; frequent your favorite fast-food restaurant; have a candy bar. Whatever you heart desires, feel free to indulge.

The refeed day serves a dual purpose. For one, it helps to maintain dietary adherence. The biggest diet-related fear most people have is that they'll never again be able to enjoy their favorite foods. This is often their downfall. After several months of deprivation, they break down and go on an eating binge, scarfing down everything in sight. And once you start bingeing, chances are that you'll abandon your diet altogether.

However, by allowing you to satisfy all your cravings, the refeed quashes temptation. You won't feel food-deprived, making dieting a much more palatable (no pun intended!) experience. And when you are content with your diet, there's less of a tendency to binge out, translating into better results.

In addition to providing a psychological boost, the refeed also confers distinct physiological benefits. Specifically, it helps you to avoid reaching a dietary plateau. This has to do with a phenomenon called *set point*. Simply stated, set point is the body's way of physiologically regulating your weight. Through various internal processes, there is a coordinated effort by your body to adjust the intake and expenditure of energy so that a specified amount of fat stores are maintained. Any attempt to deviate from this predetermined level is actively resisted.

Researchers theorize that your set point is imprinted while you're in your mother's womb. From the moment you are conceived, nature is at work deciding how much fat your body will strive to maintain. This process is unique to each individual. One person might have a set point of, say, 10 percent body fat while another might have one of 30 percent. The exact number is, for the most part, dependent on the genes of your parents.

Your set point can be traced back to the dawn of humanity. During Paleolithic times, there were no supermarkets or grocery stores that conveniently stocked an assortment of your favorite goodies. If you wanted to eat, you had to be proactive and hunt or scavenge for your food. Humans chased down wild game with primitive implements and scavenged the land for nuts and berries.

Unfortunately, there were prolonged periods where food was scarce, especially during the winter months. Days or even weeks could go by without having a meal. To deal with these continual feast-or-famine cycles, the human body developed an affinity to store energy (in the form of body fat) when it was available and then use the fat reserves for fuel during periods of deprivation. This generally followed a seasonal pattern. Our ancestors would fatten up during the warm summer months when there was an abundance of food so that they would have enough stored energy to endure the frigid winter months when food was scarce.

The problem with overly strict diets is that they make your body think it's starving. So what does your body do? Perceiving a threat to its survival, it initiates a starvation response. Through various hormonal processes—the primary hormone being *leptin* (see below)—the body slows metabolism and increases hunger to maintain ample levels of body fat. Ultimately, this leads to a weight-loss plateau, where shedding additional fat stores is all but impossible.

Understanding Leptin

Leptin is the master hormone governing body weight set point. It acts as the body's internal fat thermostat—a lipostat, if you will—that continually monitors how much fat you have and then relays this information to your brain for processing. Although there are other hormonal regulators of body weight (among them, insulin and ghrelin), none compare to leptin in terms of their long-term effects on gaining or losing fat stores.

Leptin is actually produced primarily by your fat cells, where it is secreted into the bloodstream for entry into the brain. There, a pea-sized part of the brain called the hypothalamus reads its signal and communicates with other brain centers. These brain centers then compare the amount of fat that you have with the amount of fat you are programmed to have (i.e., your set point) and make adjustments to both appetite and metabolic rate. A decrease in leptin (associated with a loss of body fat) jacks up appetite and suppresses metabolism while an increase in leptin (associated with gains in body fat) curbs appetite and elevates metabolism. In this way, body weight is maintained within a fairly narrow range of your set point.

Here's an example of how the actions of leptin translate into practice. Let's say you employ a typical calorie-restricted meal plan to get down from 20 percent body fat to 12 percent body fat. Initially, you will lose weight readily. But as you continue to diet, your body will gradually initiate the starvation response. In turn, leptin levels will fall precipitously, setting off a chain of hormonal and neurochemical events that result in an increase in appetite and a reduction in energy expenditure. The more fat you lose, the more leptin levels will fall. Consequently, if you reach your 12 percent goal and want to maintain this new weight, a great deal of resolve will be required to fight off your body's attempt to return to its set point. It's the main reason why 95 percent of all dieters fail in their quest to sustain weight loss over the long haul.

The refeed day is designed to short-circuit the starvation response. In effect, it "tricks" your body into thinking it isn't starving, allowing for the continued loss of body fat over time.

The primary means by which the refeed exerts its effects is by positively influencing leptin levels. Although leptin's main function is the control of long-term weight maintenance, it also plays a role in monitoring short-term changes in food consumption. Although leptin doesn't by itself lead to the termination of a meal, it does function locally in the stomach, increasing during periods of overfeeding and decreasing during periods of underfeeding. Jack up caloric intake for a day and leptin production skyrockets, elevating metabolism and keeping hunger at bay for a prolonged period.

To heighten the refeed's beneficial effects on leptin, it's advisable to eat a good portion of calories from carb-based foods (particularly nonfibrous starches). Glucose, one of the constituents of starch, increases leptin production much more so than fatty foods. Pasta, rice, breads, and other starches make excellent choices for the refeed. Even simple sugars such as cookies and cakes are fine. It's one of the few times that high-glycemic foods are actually desirable.

Ideally, you should keep the total calories on your refeed to about 150 percent of maintenance calories. For instance, if your maintenance intake is 1,800 calories, don't exceed 2,700 calories or so. This will give you plenty of leeway to satisfy your cravings and rev up leptin production while still keeping caloric intake within a reasonable range. Although a little bit of planned overindulgence is desirable, consuming mass quantities of food is likely to impair body composition (as well as make you pretty sick!).

For most people, refeeding once a week is all that's needed to re-regulate leptin and stave off the starvation response. At low levels of body fat, however, it can be beneficial to schedule refeeds even more frequently. You see, the lower you get under your set point, the greater your body's attempt to resist additional weight loss by shutting down leptin production. Thus, as your body fat gets down below 12 percent, refeeding every five to six days may be necessary to further your results.

It is essential, however, that you strictly adhere to your diet the rest of the week. Don't allow cheating to become a habit. Make your refeed day a planned event—a "reward" for sticking to your diet. In this way, you'll satisfy cravings and regulate leptin without triggering excess weight gain. Provided you remain regimented to the protocol, your body will become amenable to maintaining a reduced weight and you can get leaner than you previously thought possible.

Caloric Cycling

An effective technique for achieving super-low body fat levels is to stagger caloric intake—a concept called *caloric cycling*. I've used this strategy extensively when working with elite fitness competitors, but it can be equally effective for general fat-loss goals—provided you're willing to put in the effort to chart a daily schedule of your caloric intake.

Caloric cycling takes the refeed concept one step further. It involves varying the amount of calories consumed from one day to the next while keeping total calories steady over time. When properly integrated, your body is never given a chance to perceive starvation, helping to keep leptin levels consistently high.

For most women, a three-day rotation of staggered 300-calorie increments works well. For example, let's say your target caloric level is 1,500 calories a day. A three-day cycle would begin with consuming 1,200 calories on Day 1, upping that to 1,500 calories on Day 2, and then increasing to 1,800 calories on Day 3. The cycle would then repeat in similar fashion over ensuing three-day periods, continuing indefinitely throughout the course of the diet. As you can see, you'll still average 1,500 calories a day, but the higher calories trick your body into a state of satiety. If desired, you can experiment with slightly higher increments of up to about 500 calories. This can push leptin levels even higher, but the corresponding lower-calorie days can be difficult to endure.

Once you get down to your ideal body-fat level, you'll need to increase calories to a maintenance level. Maintenance involves keeping caloric intake in balance with caloric expenditure. A good way to estimate caloric intake for maintenance is to multiply your current weight by 14. Thus, if you weigh 120 pounds, your approximate caloric intake should be about 1,680 calories. As with any nutritional formula, though, this is only an estimate and some degree of adjustment in total calories might be necessary to reflect your individual body requirements and activity levels.

When coming off a weight-loss diet, it is best to increase calories incrementally until you reach maintenance level. This allows your body to slowly acclimate to the new caloric level and prevent any reactive hormonal fluctuations from interfering with metabolism or appetite. A good rule of thumb is to add back 100 calories a week until you are at maintenance. Within about a month, you'll reach your target caloric level.

Index

About the Author

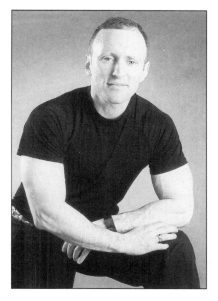

Brad Schoenfeld, CSCS, is widely regarded as one of America's leading fitness experts. He is the president of Global Fitness Services, a diverse, multifaceted fitness corporation, and he is the owner of the exclusive Personal Training Center for Women in Scarsdale, New York. Schoenfeld is a lifetime drug-free bodybuilder, who has won numerous natural bodybuilding titles including the All Natural Physique and Power Conference (ANPPC) Tri-State Naturals and USA Mixed Pairs crowns.

He is author of six fitness books, including *Sculpting Her Body Perfect* and the bestseller *Look Great Naked* (Prentice Hall Press, 2001). He is a columnist for *FitnessRX for Women* magazine, has been published or featured in virtually every major magazine (including *Cosmopolitan, Self, Marie Claire, Fitness,* and *Shape*), and has appeared on hundreds of television shows and radio programs across the United States.

Certified as a strength and conditioning specialist by the National Strength and Conditioning Association and as a personal trainer by both the American Council on Exercise and Aerobics and Fitness Association of America, Schoenfeld was awarded the distinction of master trainer by the International Association of Fitness Professionals. He is also a frequent lecturer on both the professional and consumer levels.

Schoenfeld lives in Croton-on-Hudson, New York.

Other Great Books by Brad Schoenfeld

- *Look Great Naked* (Prentice Hall Press, 2001)
- *Look Great Sleeveless* (Prentice Hall Press, 2002)
- *Sculpting Her Body Perfect* (Human Kinetics, 2002)
- *Look Great At Any Age* (Prentice Hall Press, 2003)
- *Look Great Naked Diet* (Penguin/Putnam, 2003)

Check out Brad's Web site at www.lookgreatnaked.com.

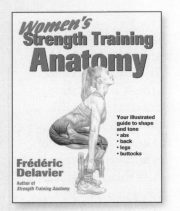
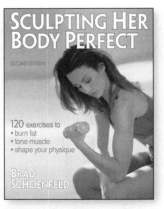
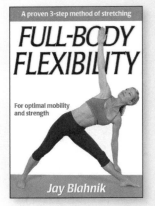
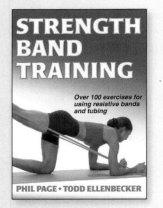
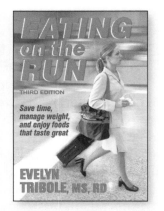
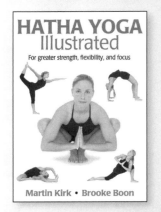
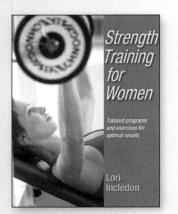